A Practical Guide to
Joint & Soft Tissue
Injection & Aspiration

A Practical Guide to

Joint & Soft Tissue
Injection & Aspiration

James W. McNabb, MD

Private Practice—Family Medicine
Piedmont HealthCare
Mooresville, North Carolina

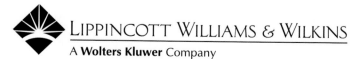

LIPPINCOTT WILLIAMS & WILKINS
A **Wolters Kluwer** Company

Philadelphia · Baltimore · New York · London
Buenos Aires · Hong Kong · Sydney · Tokyo

Acquisitions Editor: Danette Somers
Editorial Assistant: Mary Choi
Project Manager: Alicia Jackson
Senior Manufacturing Manager: Benjamin Rivera
Marketing Manager: Kathy Neely
Designer: Karen Quigley
Production Service: Nesbitt Graphics, Inc.
Printer: Quebecor World-Kingsport

Library of Congress Cataloging-in-Publication Data

McNabb, James W.
   A practical guide to joint & soft tissue injection & aspiration / James W. McNabb.
      p. ; cm.
   Includes bibliographical references and index.
   ISBN 0-7817-5363-5
 1. Joints--Diseases. 2. Musculoskeletal system--Diseases. 3. Injections,
Intra-articular. 4. Needle biopsy. 5. Aspiration and aspirators. I. Title.
II. Title: Practical guide to joint and soft tissue injection & aspiration.
   [DNLM: 1. Injections, Intra-Articular--methods. 2. Biopsy, Needle. 3.
Joint Diseases--drug therapy. WB 354 M4785p 2005]
RC932.M29 2005
616.7'2--dc22
                                                                    2004020229

10 9 8 7 6 5 4 3 2 1

This textbook is dedicated to my family.

Contents

Foreword

This text is an evidence-based guide that explains both the theory and actual performance of joint and soft tissue injections and aspirations. I hope that physicians, physician assistants, nurse practitioners, and other qualified medical providers learn these techniques to bring additional therapeutic options to patients. A common experience for many physicians is that musculoskeletal medicine was not adequately covered in our education. All too often this field is ignored in medical school and residency training in favor of topics that are more inpatient based. In addition, training in musculoskeletal medicine is frequently delegated to orthopedic surgeons who may not appreciate the extensive capabilities of primary care providers. Many of us have been taught to refer patients to these specialists if simple therapeutic measures such as the administration of NSAIDS do not bring the desired outcome. As a result, many medical providers do not know how to offer these simple yet effective therapeutic techniques to treat a variety of common musculoskeletal conditions seen routinely in primary care.

Using the techniques illustrated in this textbook can add significant clinical power to primary care medical providers. This enhances the diagnostic acumen and therapeutic confidence of the clinician. Performing the injections painlessly with therapeutic effect builds positive physician-patient relationships. It also serves to enhance the patient's experience with the healthcare system. By effectively having a musculoskeletal disorder treated without referral, the patient has an efficient medical experience at minimal cost and no added inconvenience. An additional benefit to the practitioner is that the procedural reimbursement can provide a welcome source of income in an increasingly difficult economic environment.

James W. McNabb, MD

Acknowledgments

I would like to acknowledge the following people and organizations who taught, encouraged, and helped me write this textbook; a project culminating 20 years of practice and teaching. First, I thank my wife, Liz, for her support during the writing of this book, my medical education, and years of practice and teaching. Without you I could not have done this. Thanks go to my three children—Ian, Bryce, and Caitlin—who are wonderfully understanding. In addition, they served as models for some of the photographs. The leadership and faculty at the University of Wyoming–Casper, Scottsdale HealthCare, and Cabarrus Family Practice Residency Programs were instrumental in allowing me to expand my knowledge base, develop sports medicine curricula, and build expertise in evidence-based medicine. Without the confidence of my patients, I would not have been able to achieve mastery of these techniques—for that I am privileged to serve as your family physician. I must acknowledge the opportunity to teach the Joint Injections workshops for the American Academy of Family Physicians at the annual scientific assemblies. Many thanks to family practice residents, medical students, and workshop participants for their trust and honest feedback. I extend special recognition to orthopedic surgeon, Robert Kalb, MD, who served as my injection mentor as we taught the AAFP workshops. It was a privilege to engage in sometimes spirited conversations about the performance of these procedures. Finally, a big thank you to Danette Somers, the editor of this book. Danette kept up a constant stream of encouragement and support during the long and arduous process of conceptualizing, outlining, organizing, writing, illustrating, editing, and proofing the text. To all involved and to so many more left unnamed—thank you!

Introduction and Foundation Concepts

The performance of joint and soft tissue injections and aspirations is a valuable skill that can be mastered by primary care physicians and qualified medical providers. These procedures can help relieve pain and improve function for the patient and at the same time empower the clinician. It is essential that these techniques be used thoughtfully and precisely in conjunction with making the correct diagnosis of musculoskeletal disorders. This can be quite challenging at times but is no more difficult than diagnosing and treating any of the other medical conditions that the primary care physician encounters daily. Learning how to confidently make an accurate diagnosis of musculoskeletal conditions is beyond the scope of this text. Several good sources are listed in the References.

An important concept is that aspiration and injection therapy is not an end in itself. It is only one treatment option. The withdrawal of fluid or the precise deposition of corticosteroid is a temporary measure that is generally used in conjunction with other modalities. Therapy may include rest, compression, splinting, ice, heat, ultrasound, physical therapy, or the administration of nonsteroidal antiinflammatory drugs (NSAIDS). Performing aspirations or injections is likely to result in recurrence if used without complementary treatment.

In this text, I present the following primary learning objectives:

- Describe the indications and contraindications for each procedure.
- Review the current medical literature.
- Select appropriate equipment for each injection or aspiration.
- Illustrate pertinent anatomic landmarks for each procedure.
- Demonstrate safe and effective technique.

KNOW THE ANATOMIC AREA IN THREE DIMENSIONS

The clinician must know the anatomy of each area that is selected for injection or aspiration. A thorough knowledge of the affected structures brings a deeper understanding of the pathologic process causing the patient's symptoms. It also enables the provider to develop a list of alternative diagnostic possibilities. With this knowledge, the physician is able to take the next step. He or she should be able to understand structural relationships beneath the surface of the skin. The physician is then able to think in three dimensions. While advancing the needle, the physician must "visualize" the location of the needle tip as it passes through the anatomic structures. These thought processes enable the physician to locate the needle precisely. This results in improved clinical outcomes through discrete placement of an anesthetic or cortico-steroid solution or insertion of a large-bore needle for fluid aspiration. Complications from needle trauma are minimized by avoidance of critical structures.

IDENTIFY THE LANDMARKS

For each injection or aspiration, the physician must identify the pertinent local anatomic landmarks. These landmarks are areas on the skin that represent underlying bony prominences or easily identifiable soft tissues. The landmarks are specific to each injection site. After identification, the structures should be marked with ink by using either a ballpoint ink pen or a surgical marking pen. After identifying the land-marks, the entry site for the needle is marked. Next, the site of injection is further identified by applying firm pressure to the skin with the retracted tip of a ballpoint pen. Doing this gives the clinician a visual frame of reference and standardizes the procedure from one patient to the next. No matter how much experience a physician has with a procedure, the process of marking the landmarks and entry site in ink should not be skipped. After committing the landmarks to a surface drawing, the pa-tient is instructed not to move that area of the body. Movement changes the relation-ships between the skin ink marks and the underlying anatomy.

USE COMMON SENSE AND KNOW YOUR LIMITS

As with any medical procedure, performing injections and aspirations places a great responsibility on the operator. The medical provider must consider the indications, contraindications, weight of evidence in the medical literature, expected benefits, pos-sible side effects, anticipated outcomes, diagnostic certainty, personal experience with the procedure, clinical experience, and knowledge of the patient's values before mak-ing a decision on whether or not to perform any intervention. This is a very complex process that requires thoughtful contemplation. It is imperative that the clinician use common sense and know his or her limits before performing any medical procedure. In some cases, it may be better to engage in this conversation with the patient and re-quest specialty consultation than to perform the procedure.

INDICATIONS

There are many indications to perform injections and aspirations. From a diagnostic standpoint, the introduction of local anesthetic solution into a joint may allow a more complete exam than is possible before relief of pain. Pain limits the musculoskeletal exam. Muscle spasm develops in response, and the patient may involuntarily limit the range of motion of the area examined. Providing effective pain relief can allow the clinician to adequately examine the area of concern. This is essential to determine the integrity of underlying structures including tendons, ligaments, and cartilage.

For example, a patient presents with acute traumatic shoulder pain. Upon exami-nation, she complains of moderately severe pain, holds the shoulder at her side, and is unable to demonstrate shoulder abduction because of pain. After injection of 10 ml of 1% lidocaine, the patient is able to demonstrate full range of motion including unre-stricted abduction. This indicates that there is not a complete tear of the rotator cuff structures. She may be able to continue to receive care directed by the primary medical provider without specialty referral at that time.

Fluid recovered by needle aspiration should be examined by the operator and considered for further laboratory analysis. Notation should be made of the fluid's color, clarity, and viscosity. Normal fluid is clear and transparent with high viscosity. The fluid may contain blood, which indicates a hemorrhagic cause—most commonly acute trauma. The fluid may also be yellow because of xanthochromia from the breakdown of hemoglobin leaking from inflamed synovium. The clarity of the fluid may be altered by the presence of white blood cells (WBCs). Less commonly, crystals and cellular debris can decrease clarity. The "string test" should be done, noting the length of descent of a "string" of synovial fluid as a single drop is slowly expressed from the needle. A string shorter than the normal 10 cm indicates abnormally thin viscosity of the fluid. Strong consideration should be given to evaluation for WBC count and differential. Microscopic examination of the fluid using polarized light may reveal the presence of crystals. Uric acid crystals diagnostic of gout are thin and needlelike and display negative birefringence, whereas calcium pyrophosphate crystals indicating pseudogout are rhomboid and short and show weak positive birefringence. Other substances that can form crystals include calcium oxalate, cholesterol, and hydroxyapatite. Bacteria seen on Gram's stain and recovered by culture confirms an infectious cause.

Therapeutically, there are many reasons to perform injections and aspirations. Removal of fluid from a joint alone can result in significant pain relief and restore joint range of motion. With relatively small joints such as the elbow, this can occur with removal of 5 or 10 ml, whereas with the knee, it is not uncommon for one to remove upwards of 100 ml or even 150 ml in chronic conditions!

Indications for therapeutic injections include effusions of unknown origin, crystalloid arthropathies, synovitis, inflammatory arthritis, osteoarthritis, and osteoarthrosis. Soft tissue indications include bursitis, tendonitis, tendinosis, epicondylitis, trigger points, ganglion cysts, neuromas, nerve entrapment syndromes, and fasciitis. With inflammatory joint and soft tissue conditions, therapeutic effect is achieved by the precise placement of a corticosteroid or local anesthetic mixture.

CONTRAINDICATIONS

While knowing the indications of aspirations and injections is important, it is perhaps even more valuable to acknowledge the situations in which these procedures are contraindicated. Absolute contraindications include performing a procedure on an uncooperative patient, lack of informed consent, history of true allergy to the proposed injected medication, previous documented severe steroid flare, injection through infected tissues, and injection of corticosteroid into critical weight-bearing tendons. In particular, the injection of steroid into and around the Achilles and patellar tendons may result in catastrophic rupture of these structures. Recovery from such rupture is often difficult, prolonged, and incomplete.

Many relative contraindications exist. These are variable and may apply only to certain patients or situations. Some of these include injections near critical structures such as arteries, veins, nerves, or pleural surfaces. Caution must be exercised in patients with coagulation disorders, allergy to the preservative in the injected solution, immunocompromised states, brittle diabetes, history of avascular necrosis, previous joint replacement at the injection site, and excessive anxiety concerning the procedure and in patients who may not follow postprocedure instructions.

Patients taking the oral anticoagulant medication warfarin do not represent an absolute contraindication to injection or aspiration. Thumboo et al. in 1998 reported in *Arthritis and Rheumatism* the results of a prospective cohort study of 32 joint and soft tissue injections and aspirations involving patients who were attending a rheumatology clinic and were taking warfarin with an international normalized ration (INR) less than 4.5. Patients followed for four weeks after the procedure showed no significant hemorrhages.

SAFETY

To ensure patient and operator safety, the following procedures should be used. First, define the local anatomic landmarks. This assures the provider that the needle is being advanced with knowledge of the underlying structures. Next, always use universal precautions to avoid inadvertent contact with sharp objects and all blood or body fluids. In order to decrease the chance of needle stick injury, there are a variety of new safe-sharp needle systems available for use. It is the practitioner's responsibility to utilize one of these designs to avoid injury and maintain compliance with OSHA regulations. Finally, always use sterile technique when performing invasive procedures on any patient.

Using sterile technique does not mean that the procedure needs to be done in an operating room environment. It does require, however, that the provider take the necessary precautions to ensure there is no chance that infectious organisms are carried into the tissues by the needle. When performing injections and aspirations follow the no-touch technique.

The no-touch technique does not allow contact of the injection site after sterile preparation of the skin. After the local landmarks are identified, the injection site is marked with ink. Then, an impression in the skin is made at that site by applying firm pressure with the retracted tip of a ballpoint pen. Next, the injection site is cleansed with alcohol and followed with providone iodine. The providone iodine solution is allowed to dry. After these steps, there is no further contact or touching of the site with any nonsterile objects. The only object that comes into contact with this site is the sterile needle followed by sterile gauze and a sterile adhesive dressing. If this technique is strictly followed, then it is unnecessary to use expensive sterile gloves, drapes, gowns, or masks while performing these procedures.

Always attempt to aspirate before injecting any substance. This confirms that the needle tip is not inside a blood vessel. This simple maneuver ensures that inadvertent intravascular injection of the injection solution does not occur.

Place the injection *within* a joint or bursa and *around* a tendon. An injection into the substance of a tendon is likely to weaken that structure. Rupture may follow, especially if it is a weight-bearing tendon such as the Achilles or patellar tendons. Avoid injection directly into nerves. Such an injection will be evident as the patient should report pain, paresthesias, or numbness at the time of needle contact with a nerve. In this case, simply withdraw the needle slightly and attempt to reposition the needle before injecting the corticosteroid solution.

After injection, the patient should remain in the office for at least 20 minutes. During this time, the office staff observes the patient for any signs of systemic or local reactions.

LOCAL ANESTHESIA

Providing the patient with a pain-free experience is the responsibility of the primary care provider. In select injections, such as the posterior approach to the subacromial space, techniques such as stretching and pinching the skin may give adequate distraction to the patient so that the pain from needle insertion is not felt.

Local anesthesia to needle introduction can be achieved by use of either topical or injectable local anesthetic agents. A vapocoolant spray such as ethyl chloride may be used to give rapid onset of brief but effective skin numbness. It is a topical skin refrigerant that causes a brief period of freezing of the epidermis. This provides several seconds of local anesthetic effect that blocks the pain associated with needle injections. To administer ethyl chloride, the bottle is held upside down approximately 12 inches from the treatment area. A stream is directed continuously on the injection site. After about 20 seconds, freezing occurs indicated by frosting of the skin. The needle is then immediately inserted into the skin, as the local anesthetic effect is brief. Care must be used as this product is flammable and damages the vinyl covering used to upholster examination tables. Chucks pads used during injections effectively keep the fluid from contact with the vinyl.

The injection of local anesthetic into joints or soft tissues serves several purposes. Administration of the local anesthetic provides short-term pain relief. This allows for patient feedback. It may provide a more comprehensive examination of the affected area without the limitation of pain. In general, a local anesthetic is mixed in the same syringe as the corticosteroid solution. The added volume of the local anesthetic helps to dilute the corticosteroid. This enables dispersion of steroid in a large joint space or bursa. Pain relief following injection confirms the proper placement of corticosteroid both to the clinician and the patient. Although pain may return after the anesthetic wears off, the patient can be assured that the injected corticosteroid should begin to exert its clinical effect after 24 to 48 hours.

There are a couple of local anesthetic choices. Most commonly, lidocaine is used. Lidocaine for local anesthetic injection is commercially available as 0.5%, 1%, and 2% concentrations. It is available with or without epinephrine. For joint and soft tissue injections I exclusively use 1% lidocaine without epinephrine. This is commonly available in 50 ml multiuse bottles containing the preservative methylparaben. Lidocaine is also available as 2 ml single-use, preservative-free vials. The 2% solution of lidocaine confers no clinically important advantage and increases the risk of toxicity following administration of large amounts. The inclusion of epinephrine likewise offers no clinical advantages and is not used in these procedures to dilute the corticosteroid. The only time that I use 1% lidocaine with epinephrine with these procedures is when providing local anesthesia before a knee aspiration and/or injection.

Bupivacaine (Marcaine, Sensorcaine) is another commonly used local anesthetic. It has a longer onset of action but offers extended anesthetic effect. It affords 6 to 8 hours of local anesthesia. Multiuse vials also contain 1 mg of methylparaben as a preservative. Many physicians prefer to mix lidocaine with 0.25% bupivacaine to give the patient rapid onset of local anesthesia with an extended duration. There is, however, no proven clinical benefit using this approach. In fact, the use of this combination may increase the chance of contamination and needle stick injury and may give the patient a false sense of security. Because the negative feedback from pain is absent for an extended period of time, the patient might suffer further injury through inadvertent use of the affected body area.

The pH of local anesthetics can be buffered to decrease local pain. The pH of 1% lidocaine without epinephrine is 6.5, while the pH of 1% lidocaine with epinephrine is 4.5. Bupivacaine is isotonic. Adding sterile sodium bicarbonate to lidocaine with epinephrine at a 1:10 ratio neutralizes the mixture and has been shown to provide significant pain relief. This is, however, not a clinically important issue with joint injections because plain lidocaine is used, not lidocaine with epinephrine.

CORTICOSTEROIDS

Corticosteroids for injection purposes are synthetic derivatives of hydrocortisone. Because these compounds reduce pain and swelling, they are commonly injected into inflamed joints and soft tissues for therapeutic effect. The exact mechanism of action of corticosteroids is complex with various sites of action. They bind to glucocorticoid receptors regulating gene transcription. There is a vascular stabilizing effect by inhibition of endothelial expression of adhesion molecules for neutrophils. Capillary dilation and vascular permeability is reduced. By altering the effect of protein synthesis, corticosteroids also reduce cytokines and other inflammatory mediators. There also is a decline in the number of macrophage and polymorphonuclear cells that migrate into the area. The end effect is reduction of inflammation resulting in a reduction of swelling and pain.

Several different corticosteroids are commercially available to use for joint and soft tissue injections (Table 1). These include triamcinolone acetonide (Kenalog), triamcinolone diacetate (Aristocort), triamcinolone hexacetonide (Aristospan), methylprednisolone acetate (Depo-Medrol), betamethasone sodium phosphate and acetate (Celestone), and dexamethasone acetate (Decadron LA). Different products have varying effects and solubility in the tissues. The solubility is inversely proportional to the biologic duration of effect of the agent. Hydrocortisone is rarely used because of its high solubility and short duration of action. It also has significant mineralocorticoid activity the other agents do not. No studies have been done that conclusively determine which corticosteroid is preferred for injection of joints or soft tissues. Without good data, the selection of the particular corticosteroid agent is left to the preference of the individual clinician. Considering medication availability, cost, and experience, I prefer to use triamcinolone acetonide (40 mg/ml). If another corticosteroid is chosen, then the equivalent dosage and volume of administration may be calculated from the comparison table (Table 2).

In general, the number of corticosteroid injections should be limited to no more often than four injections per year. This prevents the systemic complication of hypothalamic-

TABLE 1

Properties of Injectable Corticosteroids

Corticosteroid	Relative Antiinflammatory Potency	Solubility	Biological Half-life
Hydrocortisone	1	High	8–12 h
Triamcinolone (Kenalog)	5	Intermediate	12–36 h
Methylprednisolone (Depo-Medrol)	5	Intermediate	12–36 h
Betamethasone (Celestone Soluspan)	20–30	Low	26–54 h
Dexamethasone (Decadron LA)	20–30	Low	26–54 h

TABLE 2

Equivalent Dosages of Injectable Corticosteroids

Corticosteroid Preparation	Equivalent Dose/Volume
Kenalog	40 mg/ml
Depo-Medrol	40 mg/ml
Celestone Soluspan	6 mg/ml
Decadron LA	4 mg/ml

pituitary-adrenal axis suppression, osteoporosis, and local articular degradation. Table 2 presents equivalent dosages of corticosteroids used for injection. For the purposes of this book, all doses are expressed in milligrams of triamcinolone suspension (Kenalog). If the physician chooses to use another steroid, then the comparative dosage can be calculated from the table. For instance, if the text indicates that 20 mg of triamcinolone is to be used for injection into the acromioclavicular joint, then one could use either 20 mg of Kenalog, 20 mg of Depo-Medrol, 3 mg of Celestone Soluspan, or 2 mg of Decadron LA (Table 1).

VISCOSUPPLEMENTATION

The concentration and size of endogenous hyaluronan is reduced in osteoarthritis. Hyaluronan (sodium hyaluronate) is a natural complex sugar of the glycosaminoglycan family. Currently, there are three products available for injection that can be used to supplement this substance in joint fluid. These commercial agents are high-molecular-weight derivatives of hyaluronan, which is synthetically derived from rooster combs. The exact mechanism of action of viscosupplementation is unknown but may involve physical cushioning of the knee joint, antiinflammatory action, and/or the stimulation of production of endogenous hyaluronan by synoviocytes.

Injectable hyaluronan is commercially available as the products Hyalgan (Sanofi-Synthelabo), Supartz (Smith and Nephew), and Synvisc (Genzyme). They are actually classified as medical devices by the U.S. Food and Drug Administration. These agents are only approved for the treatment of pain in osteoarthritis of the knee in patients who have failed to respond adequately to conservative nonpharmacologic therapy and simple analgesics, such as acetaminophen. The safety and effectiveness of the use of Hyalgan, Supartz, or Synvisc in other joints has not been established.

Evidence-based support in the medical literature for the use of hyaluronan derivatives is incomplete. The most optimistic studies show clinical improvement up to one year following injection. However, there may be specific utility when treating patients who have brittle diabetes mellitus, those who have failed corticosteroid injections, patients who have received frequent corticosteroids and are in danger of the significant side effects from repeated administration, or those patients who have a rare allergy to corticosteroids or have developed steroid flare. Use of injected hyaluronan may allow appropriate postponement of total knee replacement surgery.

Although these products are similar, Synvisc is given intraarticularly as a series of three weekly injections. Both Hyalgan and Supartz are administered in a series of five injections at weekly intervals. All three preparations are prepackaged in sterile syringes. They are very expensive, and knowledge of the reimbursement process is recommended.

The most commonly reported adverse reactions are transient local pain, swelling, effusion of the injected knee, and rash. Administration is contraindicated in patients with allergies to avian proteins, feathers, or egg products or in patients with known hypersensitivity to hyaluronan products.

EQUIPMENT

Medical providers should organize the equipment needed to perform injections and aspirations. This should be done well before the procedure is to be performed. A dedicated cabinet can be used in a treatment room. Alternatively, an injection tray or cart can be used. Organizing all equipment in such a manner presents the materials conveniently to the practitioner (Fig. 1). This decreases the amount of time required to gather all of the necessary items. It also reduces the possibility of inadvertent medical error.

The items that should be collected include the following:

- Gloves—regular nonsterile exam gloves
- Ball point pen and/or skin marking pen
- Chucks pads—nonsterile
- Alcohol pads
- Providone iodine pads
- Gauze pads
- Adhesive bandages
- Hemostat surgical clamp
- Syringes:
  - 3 ml
  - 5 ml

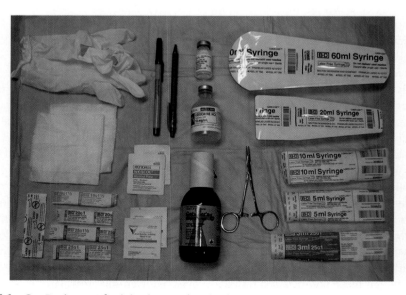

FIGURE 1 ● Equipment for injections and aspirations

- 10 ml
- 20 ml
- 60 ml
- Needles:
  - 20-gauge, 1 inch—for drawing medications and aspiration of small joints
  - 18-gauge, 1-1/2 inch—for aspiration of large joints and bursa
  - 25-gauge, 1 and 1-1/2 inch—for injections
  - 25-gauge, 3-1/2 inch spinal needles—for deep injections (rarely used)
- Ethyl chloride vapocoolant spray
- Lidocaine, 1% plain
- Lidocaine 1% with epinephrine—for local anesthesia when performing knee aspirations
- Steroid of choice (triamcinolone 40 mg/ml)
- Viscosupplementation agent of choice—ordered as needed

TECHNIQUE

When performing injections and/or aspirations, the medical provider must follow a standardized routine. This helps organize the clinician, prepares the patient, and reduces the possibility of procedural omissions. The following steps should be done in the order presented:

1. Determine the medical diagnosis and consider relevant differential diagnoses.
2. Discuss the proposed procedure and alternatives with the patient.
3. Obtain informed consent from the patient.
4. Collect and prepare required materials.
5. Identify and mark the anatomic landmarks and injection site with ink. Do not allow the patient to move the affected area from the time that the marks are placed until after the procedure is completed.
6. Press firmly on the skin with the retracted tip of a ballpoint pen to further identify the injection site.
7. Prepare the site for injection by cleansing of alcohol followed by application of providone iodine. Allow the providone to dry for full antibacterial effect.
8. Provide local anesthesia as indicated through use of tactile distraction, vapocoolant spray (ethyl chloride), and/or injected local anesthesia.
9. Using the no-touch technique, introduce the needle at the injection site and advance it precisely into the treatment area.
10. Aspirate fluid (optional) and send for laboratory examination if indicated. If injecting corticosteroid immediately following aspiration, do not remove the needle from the joint or bursa. In this case, grasp the needle hub firmly with a hemostat clamp, twist off the original syringe, and then immediately attach the second syringe that contains the corticosteroid.
11. Inject corticosteroid solution into the treatment area. Always aspirate before injection to avoid intravascular administration. Do not inject the medication against resistance.
12. Withdraw the needle.
13. Apply direct pressure over the injection site with a sterile gauze pad.
14. Apply an adhesive dressing.
15. Provide the patient with specific postinjection instructions.

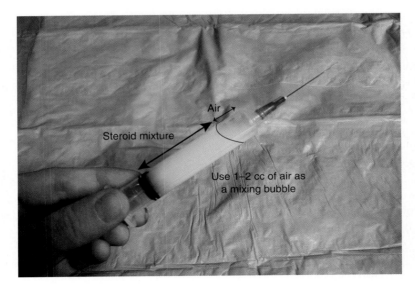

FIGURE 2 ● Mixing bubble

There is a common misconception that distributing the corticosteroid over a wide area enhances the effect from soft tissue injections. Practitioners frequently use a "fanning" or "peppering" technique to distribute the solution across the area of involvement. This, however, is frequently unnecessary. The solution, injected as a bolus, passively moves in the tendon sheaths and local fascial planes. Consideration may be given to "fanning" when injecting back muscle trigger points and trochanteric bursitis.

When injecting a corticosteroid–local anesthetic mixture, a common observation is that the corticosteroid often precipitates toward the bottom of the syringe. One way to deal with this is to draw the volume of anesthetic into the syringe followed by the corticosteroid solution. Next, 1 ml of air is aspirated into the syringe creating a "mixing bubble." Immediately before the corticosteroid–local anesthetic mixture is injected, the syringe is rapidly rotated to disperse the corticosteroid solution evenly throughout the syringe. The needle of the syringe is then pointed upwards and the small volume of air expelled before the needle is inserted into the skin (Fig. 2).

COMPLICATIONS

Complications from injections and aspirations fall into two categories—systemic and local. Systemic complications include vasovagal reactions, lidocaine allergy, lidocaine toxicity, cardiac arrhythmias, seizures, flushing, increased blood sugar in patients with diabetes, impaired immune response, psychological disturbances, adrenal suppression, irregular menses, abnormal vaginal bleeding, and osteoporosis. Local complications may involve bleeding, infection, osteonecrosis of juxtaarticular bone, ligament rupture, tendon rupture, subcutaneous atrophy, and skin depigmentation.

Steroid flare is a local reaction thought to be caused by the development of steroid crystals in the synovial space. The reaction occurs 6 to 24 hours following the corticosteroid injection. This is controversial, however, because an identical reaction can occur from a chemical synovitis caused by the preservative, methylparaben. Multiuse vials of plain lidocaine, lidocaine with epinephrine, and bupivacaine all contain 1 mg of methylparaben. In either case, the acute postinjection reaction can be managed by use of NSAIDS and ice application after a repeat aspiration confirms that there is no infection.

Pneumothorax has been reported as a complication of trigger point injections of back muscles. Injuries to the radial artery can occur with attempted aspiration of large volar wrist ganglion cysts.

AFTERCARE

Immediately following the aspiration and/or injection, apply pressure to the bandage covering the site. Once the provider is assured that the patient is stable and is not at risk of falling, the patient should be brought down from the exam table. Gentle massage and slow range of motion may be allowed to enable dispersion of the corticosteroid throughout the joint space or soft tissues. After discharge from the office, patients should be advised to look for and immediately report any adverse reactions. Of utmost importance is recognizing the early signs of infection; therefore, any swelling, redness, increased warmth, proximal red streaking, or fever of over 100 degrees should be reported immediately.

Patients often experience complete resolution of pain following injection with a local anesthetic. Because of pain relief and lack of negative feedback, there is an increased risk of further injury to the treated area. Patients should be informed that the initial pain relief is being provided by the injected local anesthetic and that its effect will only be temporary. In the case of plain 1% lidocaine, pain relief can be expected to last only about 1 hour. The antiinflammatory effect of the injected corticosteroid product usually has a 24–48 hour onset of action. Patients should be informed that the pain is expected to return in about an hour and decrease again in 1–2 days.

Additional instructions may be given following aspiration and/or injection. The patient might be directed to apply ice or even heat to the affected area. NSAIDS may be prescribed depending on the clinical situation. Studies have shown that immobilization of the affected area is not necessary, but reduced usage and activity modification is often helpful. A compressive elastic wrap or splint might be indicated. An aftercare patient education handout (see Appendix 2) that outlines the possible adverse reactions and specific instructions can be a useful tool.

BILLING AND CODING

To receive appropriate reimbursement, clinicians must assign the proper code(s) for the procedure(s) performed. This ensures fair reimbursement for the work done at the visit. A complete description of the procedures performed during the patient encounter must be documented in the medical record to support the level of coding. At the time of publication, the following Current Procedural Terminology (CPT) 2004 codes are used to bill for injection and aspirations:

- 20526—injection, therapeutic, carpal tunnel
- 20550—injection(s), single tendon sheath, or ligament, aponeurosis (e.g., plantar "fascia")
- 20551—injection(s), single tendon origin/insertion
- 20552—injection(s), single or multiple trigger point(s) in one to two muscles
- 20553—injection(s), trigger point(s) in three or more muscles

- 20600—arthrocentesis, aspiration and/or injection; *small* joint or bursa
- 20605—arthrocentesis, aspiration and/or injection; *intermediate* joint or bursa
- 20610—arthrocentesis, aspiration and/or injection; *major* joint or bursa
- 20612—aspiration and/or injection, ganglion cyst(s), any location
- 64450—injection, nerve block, therapeutic, other peripheral nerve or branch

CPT 2004 defines small joints as those in the fingers and toes. Temporomandibular, acromioclavicular, wrist, elbow, ankle, and olecranon bursa are defined as intermediate joints or bursa. Large structures are the glenohumeral joint, sacroiliac joint, hip joint, knee joint, and subacromial bursa.

According to their definitions, the CPT codes 20550, 20551, 20600, 20605, and 20610 are used once for each tendon, joint, or bursa injected. If more than one tendon, joint, or bursa is injected at a visit, then the codes are listed multiple times for each separate structure that is injected. In addition, the modifiers –51 or –59 are used to indicate when multiple procedures are performed. Usually –59 is used to code for multiple injections at different sites, but the specific modifier used is determined by the preference of each insurance carrier. Trigger point injection CPT codes 20552 and 20553 are used only once each session, regardless of the number of injections performed. CPT 2004 gives specific instructions when reporting multiple ganglion cyst aspirations and injections. In this case, the code 20612 is used and the modifier –59 appended.

CPT 2004 does not specifically define the proper code to be used for corticosteroid injection of either the ulnar nerve in cubital tunnel syndrome or injection of the interdigital nerves of the feet in Morton's neuroma. While most clinicians use the tendon injection codes for this, the author feels that until CPT descriptors change, the code 64450 most accurately reflects the procedure performed in these conditions.

Medicare and most insurance companies apply the multiple surgery rule when paying for multiple injections. They reimburse 100% for the first procedure, 50% for the second, and 25% for three or more procedures.

J codes are used to charge for the injected corticosteroid consumed during the procedure. Therapeutic injectable products, such as corticosteroids and viscosupplementation agents, are billed in addition to the injection administration codes. The J codes are not used for local anesthetics because their use is considered a necessary part of the procedure much like the needle and syringe. The charge is reflected as the number of units used during the procedure. For instance, the J code for Kenalog is expressed in 10-mg units. If the injection is done with 40 mg of Kenalog, then the patient is charged 4 units of J3301. The most common, current J codes used for injection are listed in Table 3.

An evaluation and management (E&M) code can be billed if the documentation of the visit supports the necessity and completeness of the evaluation. Otherwise, only the CPT code and associated J code can be used if a separate and distinct, medically necessary evaluation is not performed.

INFORMED CONSENT

As with any invasive procedure, informed consent must be obtained from the patient. For the purposes of documentation, this should be done in a written format. The patient must also have adequate opportunity to ask questions including discussion of alternative methods of diagnosis and treatment. An example of an informed consent form is included in Appendix 1.

TABLE 3

J Codes for Injectable Steroids

J Code	Material	Unit
J3301	Kenalog	10 mg
J1020	Depo-Medrol	20 mg
J1030	Depo-Medrol	40 mg
J1040	Depo-Medrol	80 mg
J0704	Celestone Soluspan	6 mg
J1094	Decadron LA	1 mg
J7320	Synvisc	16 mg
J7317	Hyalgan	20 mg

EVIDENCE-BASED MEDICINE

Intraarticular and soft tissue steroid injections are common procedures performed by primary care physicians. They have enjoyed acceptance and are frequently used to treat various musculoskeletal conditions. Although significant therapeutic efficacy is claimed from over 40 years of published research, a closer examination of the literature yields less convincing evidence of significant long-term improvement of specific measured outcomes. The available data supports short-term benefit from injected corticosteroids. There is currently insufficient quality data to provide a definitive answer on the efficacy of corticosteroid injections. Lack of discrete medical evidence, however, does not necessarily mean that these procedures are ineffective. Even gold-standard, evidence-based medicine resources such as Cochrane Reviews suffer from performing meta-analysis using studies flawed data. A notable example of high-quality, evidence-based data is a 1999 study by Dammers et al. in the *British Medical Journal* that documented significant improvement using injections of methylprednisolone in the treatment of carpal tunnel syndrome. New investigations that are methodologically sound are needed to measure outcomes of corticosteroid injections given for the treatment of specific conditions.

PEARLS

- Review and mark anatomic landmarks before aspirating or injecting.
- Visualize the anatomy and the procedure in three dimensions.
- Always use the no-touch technique.
- Aspirations: Use an 18-gauge needle for large joints or bursa, and use a 20-gauge needle for intermediate or small joints.
- Injections: Use a 25-gauge needle.

Subacromial Space Injection—Posterior Approach

Patients commonly present to the primary care clinician for evaluation of shoulder pain. Almost all shoulder disorders that can be treated by injection therapy involve the rotator cuff complex. These disorders are either primary from acute injury—usually superimposed on chronic degeneration—or secondary to impingement. Since the subacromial space encompasses the rotator cuff complex as well as the proximal aspect of the biceps tendon, it allows easy access to these structures for corticosteroid treatment. In patients with longstanding degenerative disease, the subacromial bursa commonly perforates into the glenohumeral joint, creating communication between the two structures.

The posterior approach to the subacromial space is the easiest to perform and is well accepted by patients. Because they cannot see the approaching needle, anxiety is diminished. A small-diameter needle is appropriate as this technique is only used to inject anesthetic and/or a steroid solution into the subacromial space. A large-diameter needle is not necessary because fluid does not collect in the space. The posterior approach is considered safe because there are no major arteries or nerves in the immediate path of the needle.

Indications	ICD-9 Code
Shoulder pain	719.41
Rotator cuff sprain	840.4
Rotator cuff tendonitis	726.10

Using local anesthetic without steroid, this injection can help the clinician determine the cause of vague shoulder pain. Relief of pain after the local anesthetic is injected into the space confirms the presence of subacromial pathology. This is known as the "impingement test."

Relevant Anatomy: (Fig. 1, Fig. 2)

PATIENT POSITION

- Sitting on the examination table.
- The patient's hands are folded in his or her lap. The hand of the shoulder that is not involved is placed over the hand of the shoulder that is to be injected. This allows

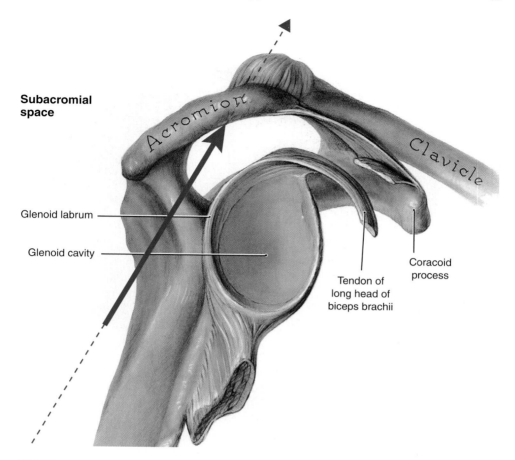

FIGURE 1 ● Right lateral shoulder (red arrow indicates path of needle). (Adapted from Agur A, Lee MJ. *Grant's Atlas of Anatomy,* 10th ed. Philadelphia: Lippincott Williams & Wilkins, 1999:456.)

consistency of positioning of the shoulder so that the landmarks do not change from the time that they are identified and marked until the time of injection.
- Once the landmarks are identified, the patient should not move the shoulder or arm.

LANDMARKS

- With the patient seated on the examination table, stand lateral and posterior to the affected shoulder.
- Find the lateral edge of the acromion and mark it with an ink pen.
- Palpate the posterior edge of the acromion and mark that.
- Having identified the posterior lateral corner of the acromion, drop a line down from that point and mark a spot 2 cm below the posterior lateral corner.
- At that site, press firmly with the retracted tip of a ballpoint pen. This indention represents the entry point for the needle.
- Next, identify the target site by placing the index finger of your nondominant hand over the superior aspect of the acromion. This will be the target for the tip of the

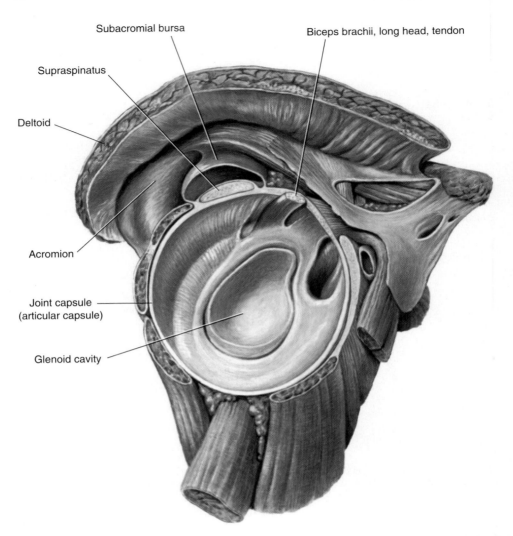

Subacromial bursa

Biceps brachii, long head, tendon

Supraspinatus

Deltoid

Acromion

Joint capsule
(articular capsule)

Glenoid cavity

FIGURE 2 ● Right lateral shoulder. (Adapted from Putz R, Pabst R. *Sobotta Atlas of Human Anatomy,* 13th ed. Philadelphia: Lippincott Williams & Wilkins, 2001:190.)

needle (Fig. 3). If your index finger is at the target site—on top of the acromion, it will be protected from accidental needle stick.

ANESTHESIA

- Local anesthesia of the skin with lidocaine or topical vapocoolant spray is not necessary in most patients.

EQUIPMENT

- 10-ml syringe
- 25-gauge, 1-1/2 inch needle. (Consider 3-1/2 inch 25-gauge needles for large individuals.)

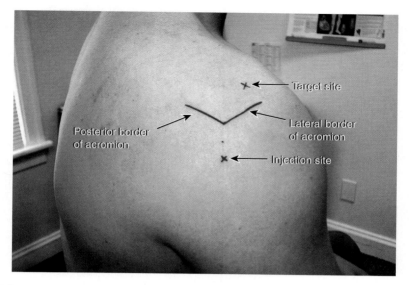

FIGURE 3 ● Right shoulder injection landmarks

- 8 ml of 1% lidocaine without epinephrine
- 1 ml of the steroid solution (40 mg of triamcinolone acetonide)
- Alcohol pads
- Betadine pads
- Sterile gauze pads
- Sterile adhesive bandage

TECHNIQUE

1. Prep the insertion site with alcohol and Betadine.
2. Using the no-touch technique, introduce the needle at the insertion site. Get underneath the acromion and advance the needle toward your target finger (Fig. 4).
3. Touch the undersurface of the acromion with the needle, back up 1–2 mm, and inject the volume of the syringe into the subacromial space. The injected solution should flow smoothly into the space. Increased resistance may indicate that the injected fluid is entering the supraspinatus muscle or tendon. In that case, advance or withdraw the needle slightly before attempting further injection.
4. Apply a sterile adhesive bandage.
5. Have the patient move the shoulder through its full range of motion. This movement distributes the steroid solution throughout the subacromial space.
6. Reexamine the shoulder after 5 minutes to confirm pain relief.

AFTERCARE

- Have the patient avoid excessive use of shoulder over the next 2 weeks.
- Consider use of an arm sling.
- Use NSAIDs, ice, and/or physical therapy as indicated.
- Consider a follow-up examination in 2 weeks.

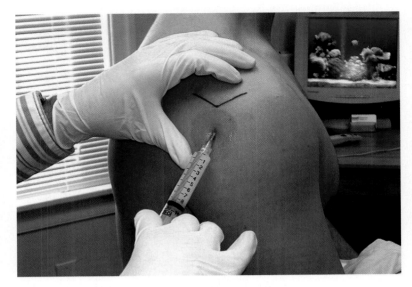

FIGURE 4 ● Right shoulder subacromial space injection

CPT code: 20610—Injection of major joint or bursa

PEARLS

- When palpating to determine the location of the acromion, use the fingertips of your index, middle, and ring fingers. Gently and methodically move in a distal to proximal direction. Mark the site where your fingers meet bone.
- Ensure that the needle is underneath the acromion before advancing it toward the target finger.
- Always keep your target finger over the acromion to protect it from accidental needle stick.

Glenohumeral Joint—
Posterior Approach

The glenohumeral joint is a relatively uncommon injection site for most primary care physicians. Successful injection can be difficult because of the limited space available in patients with adhesive capsulitis. Both anterior and posterior approaches can be used. For reasons listed in the previous chapter, the posterior approach is preferred. One uses the same injection site identified in Subacromial Space Injection—Posterior Approach. Because the long head of the biceps tendon has its origin within the joint capsule, a glenohumeral joint injection offers an approach to tendonitis of this structure.

A small-diameter needle is appropriate as this technique is only used to inject steroid solution into the joint space. A large-diameter needle is not necessary because a significant amount of fluid usually does not collect in the joint capsule.

Indications	ICD-9 Code
Shoulder pain	719.41
Shoulder adhesive capsulitis	726.0
Glenohumeral joint arthritis	716.91
Glenohumeral joint osteoarthrosis	715.91
Biceps tendonitis	726.12

Relevant Anatomy: (Fig.1, Fig. 2)

PATIENT POSITION

- Sitting on the examination table.
- The patient's hands are folded in his or her lap. This allows consistency of positioning of the shoulder so that the landmarks do not change from the time that they are identified and marked until the time of injection.
- Once the landmarks are identified, the patient should not move the shoulder or arm.

LANDMARKS

- With the patient seated on the examination table, stand lateral and posterior to the affected shoulder.
- Find the lateral edge of the acromion and mark it with an ink pen.

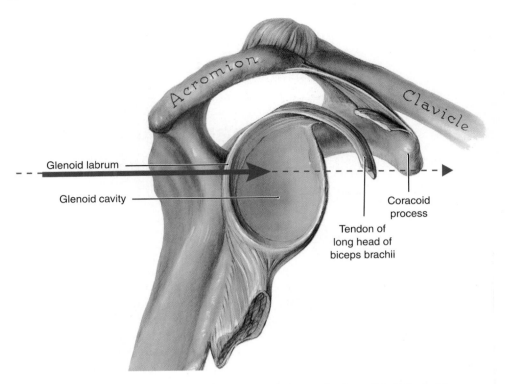

FIGURE 1 ● Right lateral shoulder (red arrow indicates path of needle). (Adapted from Agur A, Lee MJ. *Grant's Atlas of Anatomy*, 10th ed. Philadelphia: Lippincott Williams & Wilkins, 1999:456.)

- Palpate the posterior edge of the acromion and mark that.
- Having identified the posterior lateral corner of the acromion, drop a line down from that point and mark a spot 2 cm below the posterior lateral corner.
- At that site, press firmly with the retracted tip of a ballpoint pen. This indention represents the entry point for the needle.
- Next, identify the target site by placing the index finger of your nondominant hand over the coracoid process. This will be the target for the tip of the needle.

ANESTHESIA

- Local anesthesia of the skin with lidocaine or topical vapocoolant spray is not necessary in most patients.

EQUIPMENT

- 3-ml syringe
- 25-gauge, 1-1/2 inch needle. (Consider 3-1/2 inch, 25-gauge needles for large individuals.)
- 1 ml of 1% lidocaine without epinephrine
- 1 ml of the steroid solution (40 mg of triamcinolone acetonide)
- Alcohol pads

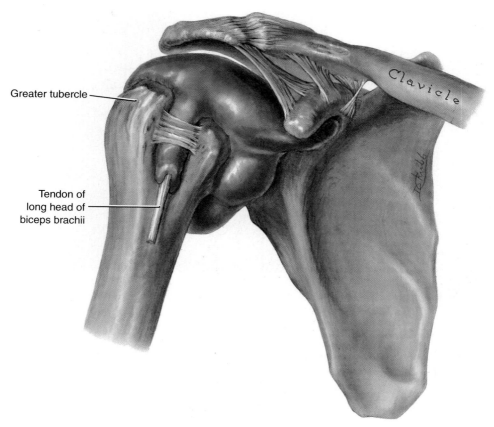

Greater tubercle

Tendon of
long head of
biceps brachii

Clavicle

FIGURE 2 ● Right lateral shoulder. (Adapted from Agur A, Lee MJ. *Grant's Atlas of Anatomy*, 10th ed. Philadelphia: Lippincott Williams & Wilkins, 1999:454.)

- Betadine pads
- Sterile gauze pads
- Sterile adhesive bandage

TECHNIQUE

1. Prep the insertion site with alcohol and Betadine.
2. Using the no-touch technique, introduce the needle at the insertion site. Advance the needle toward your target finger (Fig. 3).
3. The needle will contact the humeral head. Withdraw 1–2 mm, and inject the volume of the syringe into the glenohumeral joint. The injected solution should flow smoothly into the space. If increased resistance is encountered, advance or withdraw the needle slightly before attempting further injection.
4. Apply a sterile adhesive bandage.
5. Have the patient move the shoulder through its full range of motion. This movement distributes the steroid solution throughout the subacromial space.
6. Reexamine the shoulder after 5 minutes to confirm pain relief.

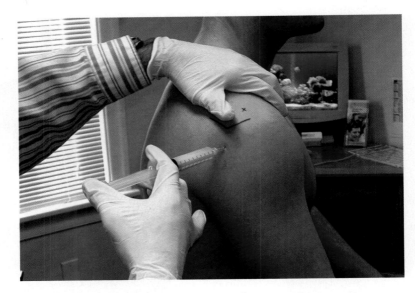

FIGURE 3 ● Glenohumeral joint injection—posterior approach

AFTERCARE

- Have the patient avoid excessive use of shoulder over the next 2 weeks.
- Consider use of an arm sling.
- Use NSAIDs, ice, and/or physical therapy as indicated.
- Consider a follow-up examination in 2 weeks.

CPT code: 20610—Injection of major joint or bursa

PEARLS

- When palpating to determine the location of the acromion, use the fingertips of your index, middle, and ring fingers. Gently and methodically move in a distal to proximal direction. Mark the site where your fingers meet bone.
  - A smaller volume of lidocaine is used in this injection compared to the subacromial space injection because the joint capsule may be stenosed—especially in patients with adhesive capsulitis.

Glenohumeral Joint— Anterior Approach

The glenohumeral joint is a relatively uncommon injection site for most primary care physicians. Successful injection can be difficult because of the limited space available in patients with adhesive capsulitis. Because the physician is operating in front of the patient, this technique generates much more patient anxiety and perceived pain. For these reasons, the posterior approach is preferred. Because the long head of the biceps tendon has its origin within the joint capsule, a glenohumeral joint injection offers an approach to tendonitis of this structure.

A small-diameter needle is appropriate as this technique is only used to inject steroid solution into the joint space. A large-diameter needle is not necessary because a significant amount of fluid usually does not collect in the joint capsule.

Indications	ICD-9 Code
Shoulder pain	719.41
Shoulder adhesive capsulitis	726.0
Glenohumeral joint arthritis	716.91
Glenohumeral joint osteoarthrosis	715.91
Biceps tendonitis	726.12

Relevant Anatomy (Fig. 1, Fig. 2)

PATIENT POSITION

- Sitting on the examination table.
- The patient's hands are folded in his or her lap. This allows consistency of positioning of the shoulder so that the landmarks do not change from the time that they are identified and marked until the time of injection.
- Once the landmarks are identified, the patient should not move the shoulder or arm.

LANDMARKS

- With the patient seated on the examination table, stand lateral and anterior to the affected shoulder.
- Identify the coracoid process. This is the hard and somewhat tender knob of bone immediately medial to the humeral head (Fig. 3).

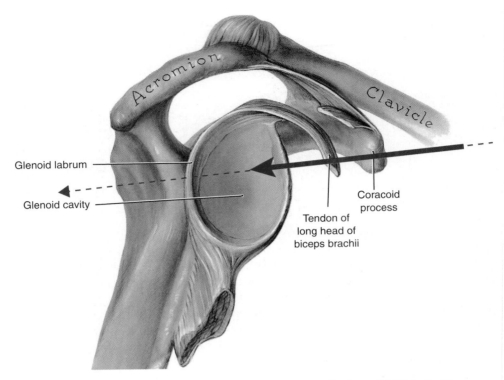

Glenoid labrum

Glenoid cavity

Coracoid process

Tendon of long head of biceps brachii

FIGURE 1 ● Right lateral shoulder (red arrow indicates path of needle). (Adapted from Agur A, Lee MJ. *Grant's Atlas of Anatomy*, 10th ed. Philadelphia: Lippincott Williams & Wilkins, 1999:456.)

- The injection point is just 1 cm lateral to the coracoid process. At that site, press firmly with the retracted tip of a ballpoint pen. This indention represents the entry point for the needle.
- Find the lateral edge of the acromion and mark it with an ink pen.
- Palpate the posterior edge of the acromion and mark that.
- Having identified the posterior lateral corner of the acromion, drop a line down from that point and mark a spot 2 cm below the posterior lateral corner. This will be the target for the tip of the needle.

ANESTHESIA

- Local anesthesia of the skin with lidocaine or topical vapocoolant spray is not necessary in most patients.

EQUIPMENT

- 3-ml syringe
- 25-gauge, 1-1/2 inch needle. (Consider longer 25-gauge needles for large individuals.)
- 1 ml of 1% lidocaine without epinephrine
- 1 ml of the steroid solution (40 mg of triamcinolone acetonide)
- Alcohol pads
- Betadine pads
- Sterile gauze pads
- Sterile adhesive bandage

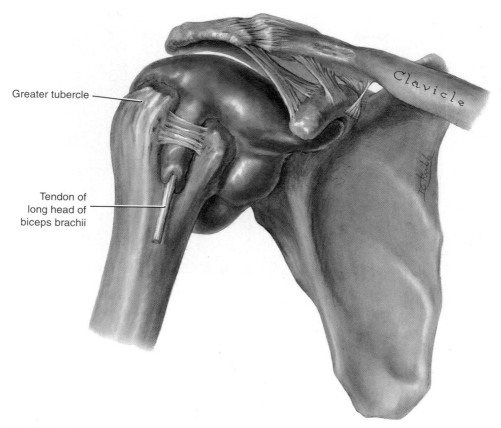

FIGURE 2 ● Right anterior shoulder showing the glenohumeral joint capsule. (Adapted from Agur A, Lee MJ. *Grant's Atlas of Anatomy*, 10th ed. Philadelphia: Lippincott Williams & Wilkins, 1999:454.)

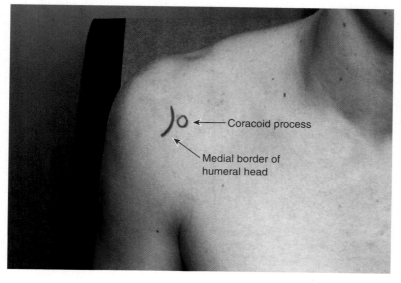

FIGURE 3 ● Anterior right shoulder landmarks

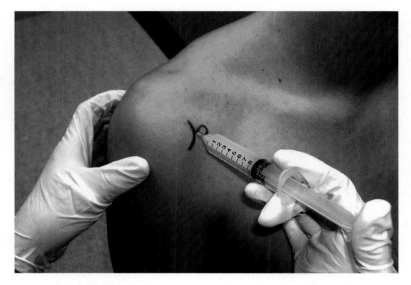

FIGURE 4 ● Glenohumeral joint injection—anterior approach

TECHNIQUE

1. Prep the insertion site with alcohol and Betadine.
2. Using the no-touch technique, introduce the needle at the insertion site. Advance the needle toward your target finger (Fig. 4).
3. The needle will contact the humeral head. Withdraw 1–2 mm and inject the volume of the syringe into the glenohumeral joint. The injected solution should flow smoothly into the space. If increased resistance is encountered advance or withdraw the needle slightly before attempting further injection.
4. Apply a sterile adhesive bandage.
5. Have the patient move the shoulder through its full range of motion. This movement distributes the steroid solution throughout the subacromial space.
6. Reexamine the shoulder after 5 minutes to confirm pain relief.

AFTERCARE

- Have the patient avoid excessive use of shoulder over the next 2 weeks.
- Consider use of an arm sling.
- Use NSAIDs, ice, and/or physical therapy as indicated.
- Consider a follow-up examination in 2 weeks.

CPT code: 20610—Injection of major joint or bursa

PEARLS

- When palpating to determine the location of the coracoid, use the fingertips of your index, middle, and ring fingers. Firmly palpate the humeral head and methodically move in a lateral to medial direction. Mark the site where your fingers meet the coracoid.

- When palpating to determine the location of the acromion, use the fingertips of your index, middle, and ring fingers. Gently and methodically move in a distal to proximal direction. Mark the site where your fingers meet bone.
- A smaller volume of lidocaine is used in this injection compared to the subacromial space injection because the joint capsule may be stenosed—especially in patients with adhesive capsulitis.

Acromioclavicular Joint

The acromioclavicular (AC) joint is a relatively uncommon injection site for most primary care physicians. Successful injection can be difficult because of the small joint space. A small-diameter needle is appropriate as this technique is only used to inject steroid solution into the AC joint.

Indications	ICD-9 Code
AC joint pain	719.41
AC joint sprain	840.0
AC joint arthritis	716.91
AC joint osteoarthrosis	715.91

Relevant Anatomy: (Fig. 1)

PATIENT POSITION

- Sitting or lying supine on the examination table.
- The patient's hands are folded in his or her lap. This allows consistency of positioning of the shoulder so that the landmarks do not change from the time that they are identified and marked until the time of injection.
- Once the landmarks are identified, the patient should not move the shoulder or arm.
- The patient should look away from the side that is being injected. This minimizes anxiety and pain perception.

LANDMARKS

- With the patient seated on the examination table, stand lateral and anterior to the affected shoulder.
- Identify the AC joint. Palpate the clavicle in a medial to lateral direction. At the lateral aspect of the clavicle, there is a small depression that will be tender in the listed indications.
- The injection point is directly over the AC joint. At that site, press firmly with the retracted tip of a ballpoint pen. This indention represents the entry point for the needle.

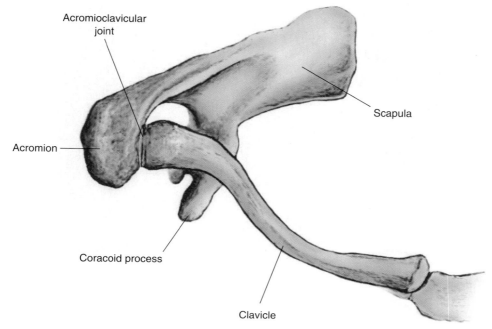

Acromioclavicular
joint

Scapula

Acromion

Coracoid process

Clavicle

FIGURE 1 ● Right acromioclavicular joint. (Adapted from Putz R, Pabst R. *Sobotta Atlas of Human Anatomy*, 13th ed. Philadelphia: Lippincott Williams & Wilkins, 2001:168.)

ANESTHESIA

• Local anesthesia of the skin with topical vapocoolant spray is preferred.

EQUIPMENT

• 3-ml syringe
• 25-gauge, 1-inch needle
• 0.5 ml of 1% lidocaine without epinephrine
• 0.5 ml of the steroid solution (20 mg of triamcinolone acetonide)
• Alcohol pads
• Betadine pads
• Sterile gauze pads
• Sterile adhesive bandage

TECHNIQUE

1. Prep the insertion site with alcohol and Betadine.
2. Achieve good topical anesthesia by using vapocoolant spray.
3. Using the no-touch technique, introduce the needle at the insertion site. Advance the needle down into the joint (Fig. 2).
4. The injected solution should flow smoothly into the space. If increased resistance is encountered advance or withdraw the needle slightly before attempting further injection.
5. Apply a sterile adhesive bandage.

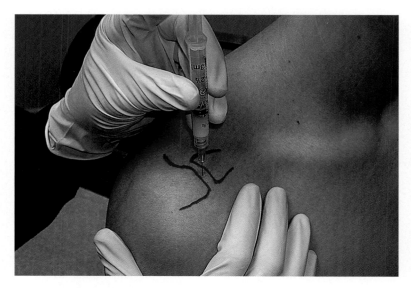

FIGURE 2 ● Acromioclavicular joint injection with landmarks

6. Have the patient move the shoulder through its full range of motion. This movement distributes the steroid solution throughout the AC joint.
7. Reexamine the shoulder after 5 minutes to confirm pain relief.

AFTERCARE

- Have the patient avoid excessive use of shoulder over the next 2 weeks.
- Consider use of an arm sling.
- Use NSAIDs, ice, and/or physical therapy as indicated.
- Consider a follow-up examination in 2 weeks.

CPT code: 20600–Injection of small joint

PEARLS

- The acromial clavicular joint is superficial. Depositing corticosteroid in the subcutaneous tissues can result in skin atrophy and hypopigmentation. Avoid the development of a subdermal wheal while performing all injections of corticosteroid
  solutions.

Sternoclavicular Joint

The sternoclavicular joint (SC) is an uncommon injection site for most primary care physicians. Successful injection can be difficult because of the small joint space. A small-diameter needle is appropriate as this technique is only used to inject steroid solution into the SC joint.

Indications	ICD-9 Code
SC joint sprain	848.41
SC joint subluxation	739.61
SC joint arthritis	716.91
SC joint osteoarthrosis	715.91

Relevant Anatomy: (Fig. 1)

PATIENT POSITION

- Supine on the examination table.
- The patient's hands are folded across his or her abdomen. This allows consistency of positioning so that the landmarks do not change from the time that they are identified and marked until the time of injection.
- Once the landmarks are identified, the patient should not move the chest, shoulder, or arm.
- The patient should look upwards and away from the side that is being injected. This minimizes anxiety and pain perception.

LANDMARKS

- Identify the SC joint. Palpate the clavicle in a lateral to medial direction. At the medial aspect of the clavicle, there is a small depression that represents the SC joint. This structure will be tender.
- It may be helpful to move the ipsilateral arm in order to more easily identify the SC joint.
- The injection point is directly over the SC joint. At that site, press firmly with the retracted tip of a ballpoint pen. This indention represents the entry point for the needle.

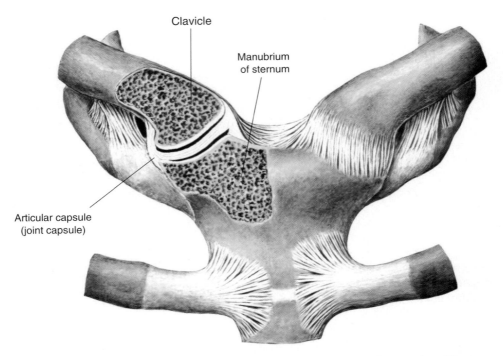

Clavicle

Manubrium
of sternum

Articular capsule
(joint capsule)

FIGURE 1 ● Sternoclavicular joint. (Adapted from Putz R, Pabst R. *Sobotta Atlas of Human Anatomy*, 13th edition. Philadelphia: Lippincott Williams & Wilkins, 2001:167.)

ANESTHESIA

• Local anesthesia of the skin with topical vapocoolant spray.

EQUIPMENT

• 3-ml syringe
• 25-gauge, 1-inch needle
• 0.5 ml of 1% lidocaine without epinephrine
• 0.5 ml of the steroid solution (20 mg of triamcinolone acetonide)
• Alcohol pads
• Betadine pads
• Sterile gauze pads
• Sterile adhesive bandage

TECHNIQUE

1. Prep the insertion site with alcohol and Betadine.
2. Achieve good topical anesthesia by using vapocoolant spray.
3. Using the no-touch technique, introduce the needle at the insertion site. Advance the needle down into the joint (Fig. 2).
4. The injected solution should flow smoothly into the space. If increased resistance is encountered advance or withdraw the needle slightly before attempting further injection.
5. Apply a sterile adhesive bandage.

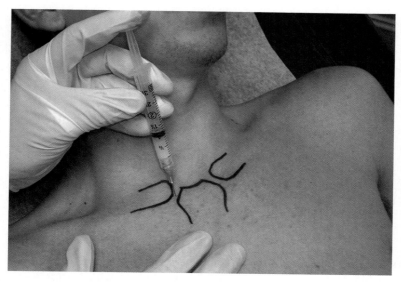

FIGURE 2 ● Sternoclavicular joint injection with landmarks

6. Have the patient move their shoulder through its full range of motion. This movement distributes the steroid solution throughout the SC joint.
7. Reexamine the shoulder in 5 minutes to confirm pain relief.

AFTERCARE

- Have the patient avoid excessive use of shoulder over the next 2 weeks.
- Consider use of an arm sling.
- Use NSAIDs, ice, and/or physical therapy as indicated.
- Consider a follow-up examination in 2 weeks.

CPT code: 20600—Injection of small joint

PEARLS

- The sternoclavicular joint is superficial. Depositing corticosteroid in the subcutaneous tissues can result in skin atrophy and hypopigmentation. Avoid the development of a subdermal wheal while performing all injections of corticosteroid solutions.

Elbow Joint

Aspiration and/or injection of the elbow joint is an uncommon procedure. Tense collections of blood from a distended elbow joint develop with fractures of the radial head. Significant pain relief follows aspiration. Arthritis in the elbow most commonly occurs as a result of rheumatoid arthritis, gout, and osteoarthritis. This may respond to corticosteroid injection.

Indications	ICD-9 Code
Elbow pain	729.5
Elbow sprain	841.9
Elbow arthritis	716.92

Relevant Anatomy: (Fig. 1)

PATIENT POSITION

- Supine on the examination table with the head of the bed elevated 30 degrees.
- The elbow is slightly flexed.
- The affected elbow may be supported by placing rolled towels underneath it.
- The wrist is in a neutral position.

LANDMARKS

- Locate the depression immediately proximal to the radial head.
- This can also be found by palpating the lateral aspect of the elbow while supinating and pronating the wrist.
- At that site, press firmly with the retracted tip of a ballpoint pen. This indention represents the entry point for the needle.

ANESTHESIA

- Local anesthesia of the skin with topical vapocoolant spray.

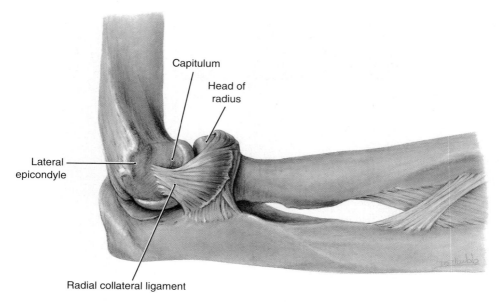

Capitulum

Head of
radius

Lateral
epicondyle

Radial collateral ligament

FIGURE 1 ● Right lateral elbow joint. (Adapted from Agur A, Lee MJ. *Grant's Atlas of Anatomy*, 10th ed. Philadelphia: Lippincott Williams & Wilkins, 1999:470.)

EQUIPMENT

- 3-ml syringe
- 10-ml syringe—for optional aspiration
- 25-gauge, 1-inch needle
- 20-gauge, 1-inch needle—for optional aspiration
- 1 ml of 1% lidocaine without epinephrine
- 1 ml of the steroid solution (40 mg of triamcinolone acetonide)
- Alcohol pads
- Betadine pads
- Sterile gauze pads
- Sterile adhesive bandage
- Nonsterile, clean chucks pad

TECHNIQUE

1. Prep the insertion site with alcohol and Betadine.
2. Achieve good topical anesthesia by using vapocoolant spray.
3. Using the no-touch technique, introduce the needle at the insertion site.
4. Advance the needle into the elbow joint. This places the needle tip between the humeral lateral condyle and the radial head (Fig. 2).
5. If aspirating, withdraw fluid using a 20-gauge, 1-inch needle with the 10-ml syringe.
6. If injection of corticosteroid is to follow the aspiration, grasp the needle firmly, remove the 10-ml syringe from the 20-gauge needle and then attach the 3-ml syringe filled with the steroid-lidocaine mixture.

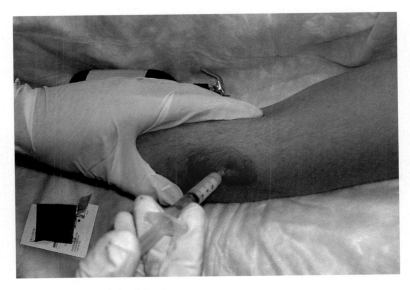

FIGURE 2 ● Left elbow joint injection

7. If only injecting the steroid mixture, use a 25-gauge, 1-inch needle with the 3-ml syringe.
8. The injected solution should flow smoothly into the space. If increased resistance is encountered, advance or withdraw the needle slightly before attempting further injection.
9. Apply a sterile adhesive bandage.
10. Have the patient move the elbow through its full range of motion. This movement distributes the steroid solution throughout the joint.
11. Reexamine the elbow after 5 minutes to confirm pain relief.

AFTERCARE

- Consider use of a neoprene elbow sleeve.
- Have the patient avoid vigorous use of the elbow over the next 2 weeks.
- Use NSAIDs, ice, and/or physical therapy as indicated.
- Consider a follow-up examination in 2 weeks.

CPT code: 20605—Arthrocentesis, aspiration, and/or injection of intermediate joint or bursa

PEARLS

- The joint space at the radial head can be "opened up" by extending the elbow.
- Because the elbow has a narrow joint space, a 20-gauge needle is used.
- If a fracture is suspected, do not inject corticosteroid.

Olecranon Bursitis

Olecranon bursitis is a relatively common aspiration and injection site for primary care physicians. Successful aspiration is usually easy because the location of the bursa is readily evident. The subcutaneous olecranon bursa may become inflamed and accumulate fluid when subjected to repeated excessive pressure or friction. The fluid may consist of blood in acute trauma, thick proteinaceous mucoid fluid after repetitive injury, or purulent fluid if infected. Corticosteroids should never be administered if an infectious bursitis is suspected.

An 18-gauge needle is used to aspirate a large volume of fluid. Occasionally the clinician may elect to inject a steroid solution if the fluid recollects—as long as an infection can be excluded.

Indications	ICD-9 Code
Olecranon bursitis	726.33

Relevant Anatomy: (Fig. 1)

PATIENT POSITION

- Supine on the examination table.
- The affected elbow is maximally flexed.
- The patient should look away from the side that is being injected. This minimizes anxiety and pain perception.

LANDMARKS

- The point of maximum fluctuance is identified.
- At that site, press firmly with the retracted tip of a ballpoint pen. This indention represents the entry point for the needle.

ANESTHESIA

- Local anesthesia of the skin with topical vapocoolant spray.

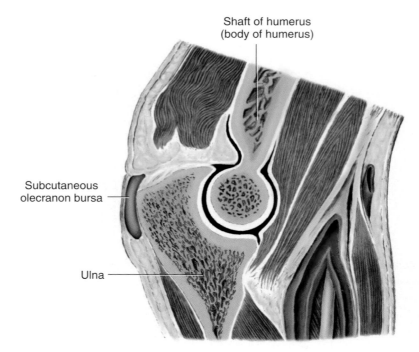

Shaft of humerus
(body of humerus)

Subcutaneous
olecranon bursa

Ulna

FIGURE 1 ● Left lateral elbow. (Adapted from Putz R, Pabst R. *Sobotta Atlas of Human Anatomy*, 13th ed. Philadelphia: Lippincott Williams & Wilkins, 2001:177.)

EQUIPMENT

- 20-ml syringe
- 3-ml syringe—for optional injection
- 18-gauge, 1-1/2 inch needle
- Hemostat—for optional injection following aspiration
- 1 ml of 1% lidocaine without epinephrine—for optional injection
- 1 ml of the steroid solution (40 mg of triamcinolone acetonide)—for optional injection
- Alcohol pads
- Betadine pads
- Sterile gauze pads
- Sterile adhesive bandage
- Nonsterile, clean chucks pad

TECHNIQUE

1. Prep the insertion site with alcohol and Betadine.
2. Achieve good topical anesthesia by using vapocoolant spray.
3. Using the no-touch technique, introduce the needle at the insertion site. Advance the needle into the center of the bursa.
4. Aspiration should be easily accomplished (Figs. 2 and 3). Use multiple syringes if the effusion is large.

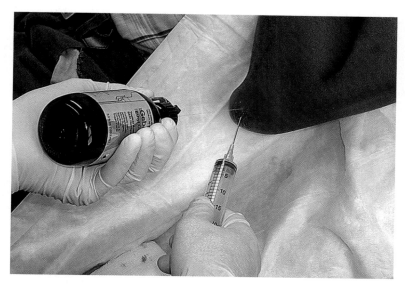

FIGURE 2 ● Left olecranon bursa aspiration

5. If injection following aspiration is elected, grasp the hub of the needle with a hemostat, remove the large syringe from the 18-gauge needle, and then attach the 3-ml syringe filled with the steroid solution.
6. The injected solution should flow smoothly into the space. If increased resistance is encountered, advance or withdraw the needle slightly before attempting further injection.
7. Apply a sterile adhesive bandage followed by a compressive elastic bandage.
8. Reexamine the elbow after 5 minutes to confirm pain relief.

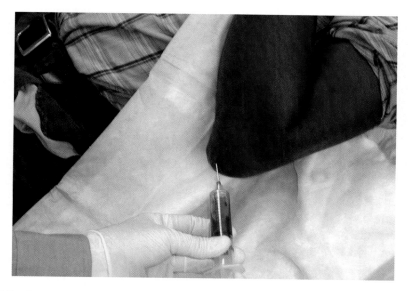

FIGURE 3 ● Aspiration of hemorrhagic olecranon bursitis

AFTERCARE

- Have the patient avoid excessive use of elbow over the next 2 weeks.
- Consider use of a neoprene elbow sleeve or elastic compression bandage.
- Use NSAIDs, ice, and/or physical therapy as indicated.
- Consider a follow-up examination in 2 weeks.

CPT code: 20605—Aspiration and/or injection of intermediate bursa

PEARLS

- If the olecranon bursitis is the result of an infection or acute hemorrhagic event, do not follow aspiration with corticosteroid injection.
- Injection of corticosteroid is usually reserved for recurrent bursitis.

Lateral Epicondylitis

Lateral epicondylitis is one of the most common soft tissue conditions treated by primary care providers. It usually is the result of an overuse injury to the origin of the wrist extensor and supinator muscle groups. Injection of corticosteroids for the treatment of lateral epicondylitis is one of the most common injections. A small-diameter needle is appropriate as there will not be a fluid collection.

Indications	ICD-9 Code
Lateral epicondylitis	726.32

Relevant Anatomy: (Fig. 1)

PATIENT POSITION

- Supine on the examination table.
- The affected elbow is slightly flexed.
- The wrist is in a neutral to slightly pronated position.

LANDMARKS

- The point of maximum tenderness over the lateral epicondyle is identified.
- At that site, press firmly with the retracted tip of a ballpoint pen. This indention represents the entry point for the needle.

ANESTHESIA

- Local anesthesia of the skin with topical vapocoolant spray.

EQUIPMENT

- 3-ml syringe
- 25-gauge, 1-inch needle
- 1 ml of 1% lidocaine without epinephrine

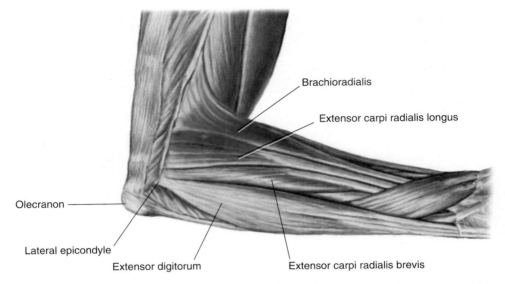

Brachioradialis

Extensor carpi radialis longus

Olecranon

Lateral epicondyle

Extensor digitorum

Extensor carpi radialis brevis

FIGURE 1 ● Right lateral elbow muscles. (Adapted from Putz R, Pabst R. *Sobotta Atlas of Human Anatomy*, 13th ed. Philadelphia: Lippincott Williams & Wilkins, 2001:187.)

- 1 ml of the steroid solution (40 mg of triamcinolone acetonide)
- Alcohol pads
- Betadine pads
- Sterile gauze pads
- Sterile adhesive bandage
- Nonsterile, clean chucks pad

TECHNIQUE

1. Prep the insertion site with alcohol and Betadine.
2. Achieve good topical anesthesia by using vapocoolant spray.
3. Using the no-touch technique, introduce the needle at the insertion site. Advance the needle to the bone of the lateral epicondyle (Fig. 2).
4. Withdraw the needle 1–2 mm.
5. Inject the steroid solution steadily into this area. If increased resistance is encountered advance or withdraw the needle slightly before attempting further injection.
6. Apply a sterile adhesive bandage followed by a compressive elastic bandage.
7. Reexamine the elbow after 5 minutes to confirm pain relief.

AFTERCARE

- Have the patient avoid excessive wrist extension over the next 2 weeks.
- Consider use of a neoprene elbow sleeve or elastic compression bandage.
- Consider the use of a wrist brace to limit wrist extension.
- Use NSAIDs, ice, heat, and/or physical therapy as indicated.
- Consider a follow-up examination in 2 weeks.

CPT code: 20551—Injection of tendon origin or insertion

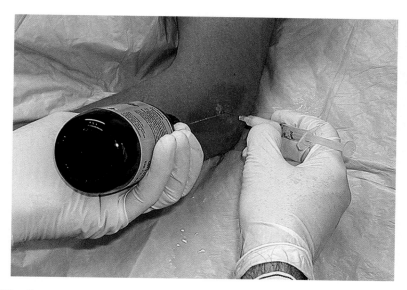

FIGURE 2 ● Left elbow lateral epicondylitis injection

PEARLS

- Entrapment of branches of the radial nerve in the elbow and forearm can mimic the pain of lateral epicondylitis. Radial tunnel syndrome is most commonly caused by entrapment of the deep radial nerve as it enters the supinator muscle at the arcade of Frohse. Pain in this condition occurs about 4 cm distal to the lateral epicondyle. Successful treatment may require surgical release.
- The lateral epicondylitis injection can be superficial—especially in thin persons. Depositing corticosteroid in the subcutaneous tissues can result in skin atrophy and

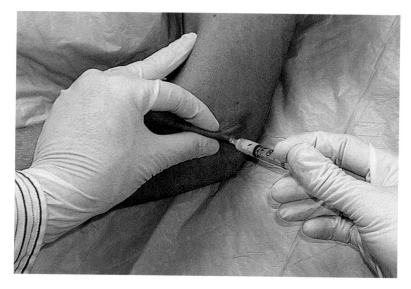

FIGURE 3 ● Pinch up tissue to avoid subcutaneous deposition

hypopigmentation. This particular injection is notorious for the development of this complication. Avoid the development of a subdermal wheal while performing all injections of corticosteroid solutions.

- To prevent this complication, use the following technique. After insertion, gently grasp the skin on either side of the needle and push that up toward the syringe. This provides a greater distance between the skin and the actual injection site, thus minimizing the chance of developing atrophy and hypopigmentation (Fig. 3).

Medial Epicondylitis

Medial epicondylitis is a fairly common soft tissue condition encountered by primary care physicians. It usually is the result of an overuse injury to the origin of the wrist flexor and pronator muscle groups. A small-diameter needle is appropriate as there will not be a fluid collection.

Indications	ICD-9 Code
Medial epicondylitis	726.31

Relevant Anatomy: (Fig. 1)

PATIENT POSITION

- Supine on the examination table.
- Upper arm at 30 degrees of abduction and full external rotation.
- The affected elbow is flexed at 90 degrees with the wrist in supination.

LANDMARKS

- The point of maximum tenderness over the medial epicondyle is identified.
- At that site, press firmly with the retracted tip of a ballpoint pen. This indention represents the entry point for the needle.

ANESTHESIA

- Local anesthesia of the skin with topical vapocoolant spray.

EQUIPMENT

- 3-ml syringe
- 25-gauge, 1-inch needle
- 1 ml of 1% lidocaine without epinephrine
- 1 ml of the steroid solution (40 mg of triamcinolone acetonide)

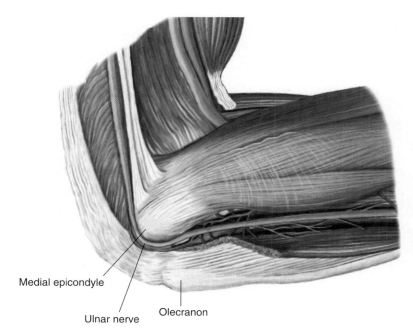

Medial epicondyle

Ulnar nerve   Olecranon

FIGURE 1 ● Left medial elbow. (Adapted from Putz R, Pabst R. *Sobotta Atlas of Human Anatomy*, 13th ed. Philadelphia: Lippincott Williams & Wilkins, 2001:241.)

- Alcohol pads
- Betadine pads
- Sterile gauze pads
- Sterile adhesive bandage
- Nonsterile, clean chucks pad

TECHNIQUE

1. Prep the insertion site with alcohol and Betadine.
2. Achieve good topical anesthesia by using vapocoolant spray.
3. Using the no-touch technique, introduce the needle at the insertion site. Advance the needle to the bone of the medial epicondyle (Fig. 2).
4. Withdraw the needle 1–2 mm.
5. Inject the steroid solution steadily into this area. If increased resistance is encountered advance or withdraw the needle slightly before attempting further injection.
6. Apply a sterile adhesive bandage followed by a compressive elastic bandage.
7. Reexamine the elbow after 5 minutes to confirm pain relief.

AFTERCARE

- Have the patient avoid excessive wrist flexion or pronation over the next 2 weeks.
- Consider use of a neoprene elbow sleeve or elastic compression bandage.
- Consider the use of a wrist brace to limit wrist flexion.
- Use NSAIDs, ice, heat, and/or physical therapy as indicated.
- Consider a follow-up examination in 2 weeks.

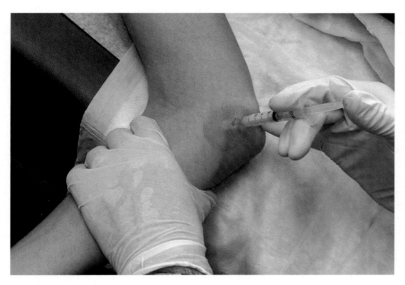

FIGURE 2 ● Right medial epicondylitis injection

CPT code: 20551—Injection of tendon origin or insertion

PEARLS

- The ulnar nerve is in close proximity to this injection. It courses just posterior and inferior to the medial epicondyle. On occasion, the local anesthetic spreading out from a properly placed injection may affect the ulnar nerve. The patient should be warned that transient numbness might occur in the lateral aspect of the hand as well as the ring and little fingers.

Cubital Tunnel Syndrome

Cubital tunnel syndrome is an uncommon condition encountered by primary care physicians. It occurs when the ulnar nerve becomes entrapped in the cubital tunnel posterior to the medial epicondyle. Treatment usually involves conservative measures including avoidance of predisposing repetitive movements, nighttime application of an elbow brace and NSAIDs. Corticosteroid injection of the cubital tunnel may bring pain relief. Care must be used to avoid injury to the ulnar nerve. Successful treatment may require surgical transposition of the nerve over the medial epicondyle.

Indications	ICD-9 Code
Cubital tunnel syndrome	354.2

Relevant Anatomy: (Fig. 1)

PATIENT POSITION

- Supine on the examination table.
- Upper arm at 30 degrees of abduction and full external rotation.
- Elbow positioned at 90 degrees of flexion.

LANDMARKS

- Identify and mark the medial epicondyle of the humerus.
- Identify and mark the course of the ulnar nerve in the ulnar groove posterior to the medial epicondyle.
- Mark the point of maximal tenderness over the ulnar nerve. This is usually just posterior to the medical epicondyle.
- At that site, press firmly with the retracted tip of a ballpoint pen. This indention represents the entry point for the needle.

ANESTHESIA

- Local anesthesia of the skin with topical vapocoolant spray.

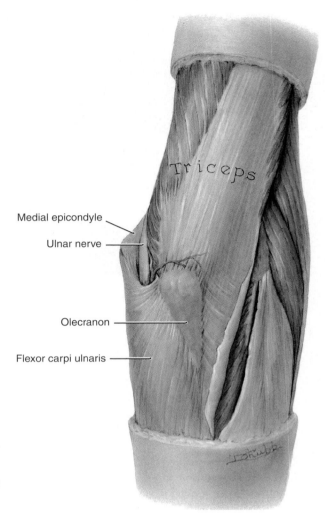

Triceps

Medial epicondyle

Ulnar nerve

Olecranon

Flexor carpi ulnaris

FIGURE 1 ● Right posterior elbow. (Adapted from Agur A, Lee MJ. *Grant's Atlas of Anatomy*, 10th ed. Philadelphia: Lippincott Williams & Wilkins, 1999:464.)

EQUIPMENT

- 3-ml syringe
- 25-gauge, 1-1/2 inch needle
- 1 ml of 1% lidocaine without epinephrine
- 1 ml of the steroid solution (40 mg of triamcinolone acetonide)
- Alcohol pads
- Betadine pads
- Sterile gauze pads
- Sterile adhesive bandage
- Nonsterile, clean chucks pad

TECHNIQUE

1. Prep the insertion site with alcohol and Betadine.
2. Achieve good topical anesthesia by using vapocoolant spray.

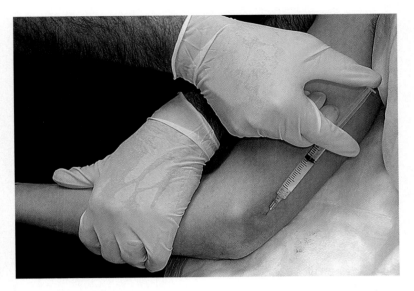

FIGURE 2 ● Right cubital tunnel injection

3. Using the no-touch technique, introduce the needle at the insertion site. Slowly advance the needle just along the side of the ulnar nerve (Fig. 2).
4. If any pain, paresthesias, or numbness is encountered, withdraw the needle slightly and redirect the needle tip at a slightly different angle.
5. When the needle is placed along the ulnar nerve, slowly deposit the steroid solution as a bolus around that structure.
6. Inject the steroid solution steadily into this area. If increased resistance is encountered advance or withdraw the needle slightly before attempting further injection.
7. Apply a sterile adhesive bandage.
8. Reexamine the elbow after 5 minutes to confirm pain relief and the development of numbness in the distribution of the ulnar nerve from the local anesthetic.

AFTERCARE

- Have the patient avoid further injury.
- Have the patient use an elbow extension brace while sleeping to avoid excessive elbow flexion.
- Use NSAIDs, ice, and/or physical therapy as indicated.
- Consider a follow-up examination in 2 weeks.

CPT code: 64450—Injection, nerve block, therapeutic, other peripheral nerve or branch

Carpal Tunnel Syndrome

Carpal tunnel syndrome is a very common condition encountered in primary care. It represents a compressive injury to the median nerve as it traverses the carpal tunnel in the wrist. This usually occurs as a result of overuse following repetitive handgrip movements or compression of the contents of the carpal tunnel from various disease processes. Predisposing factors may include injury, pregnancy, diabetes, hypothyroidism, rheumatoid arthritis, or amyloidosis. Corticosteroid injection of the carpal tunnel is an effective but underutilized treatment by primary care providers.

The specific injection technique used in this text was described by Dammers, Veering, and Vermeulan (1999). Other approaches can be used but do not have the literature references demonstrating the efficacy and safety of this approach. The study referenced is a randomized, double-blind, placebo-controlled trial. Following a single, 40-mg methylprednisone injection, there was 77% improvement at one month. It was still effective in 50% of patients at one year compared with 7% of controls. A second injection resulted in further improvement. The investigators reported no side effects.

Indications	ICD-9 Code
Carpal tunnel syndrome	354.0

Relevant Anatomy: (Fig. 1, Fig. 2)

PATIENT POSITION

- Supine on the examination table.
- The elbow is slightly flexed with the wrist in supination.
- The wrist is then positioned in slight hyperextension with the placement of chucks pads or towels underneath the supinated wrist.

LANDMARKS

- Identify and mark the distal palmar crease as shown (Fig. 3).
- Identify and mark the course of the palmaris longus and flexor carpi radialis tendons.

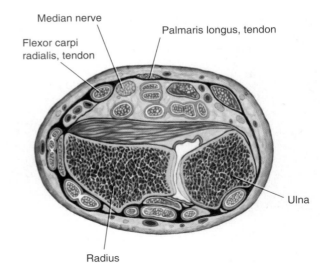

FIGURE 1 ● Right wrist cross section at the level of the distal radioulnar joint. (Adapted from Putz R, Pabst R. *Sobotta Atlas of Human Anatomy*, 13th ed. Philadelphia: Lippincott Williams & Wilkins, 2001:255.)

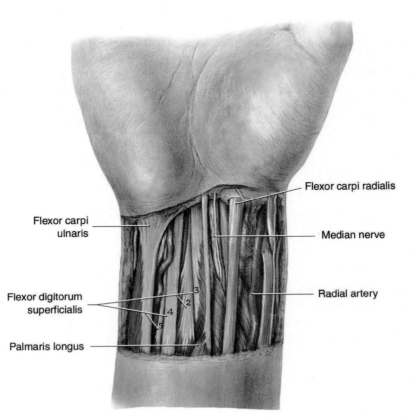

FIGURE 2 ● Right wrist—volar aspect. (Adapted from Agur A, Lee MJ. *Grant's Atlas of Anatomy*, 10th ed. Philadelphia: Lippincott Williams & Wilkins, 1999:481.)

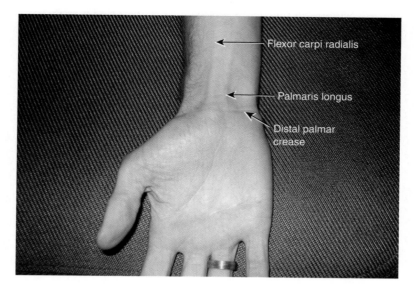

Flexor carpi radialis

Palmaris longus

Distal palmar crease

FIGURE 3 ● Right carpal tunnel surface anatomy

- Mark a spot 4 cm proximal to the distal palmar crease and between the tendons.
- At that site, press firmly with the retracted tip of a ballpoint pen. This indention represents the entry point for the needle.

ANESTHESIA

- Local anesthesia of the skin with topical vapocoolant spray.

EQUIPMENT

- 3-ml syringe
- 25-gauge, 1-1/2 inch needle
- 1 ml of 1% lidocaine without epinephrine
- 1 ml of the steroid solution (40 mg of triamcinolone acetonide)
- Alcohol pads
- Betadine pads
- Sterile gauze pads
- Sterile adhesive bandage
- Nonsterile, clean chucks pad

TECHNIQUE

1. Prep the insertion site with alcohol and Betadine.
2. Achieve good topical anesthesia by using vapocoolant spray.
3. Using the no-touch technique, introduce the needle at the insertion site. At a shallow angle of introduction, 10–20 degrees to the forearm, slowly advance the needle toward the wrist, keeping the needle between the palmaris longus and flexor carpi radialis tendons (Fig. 4).

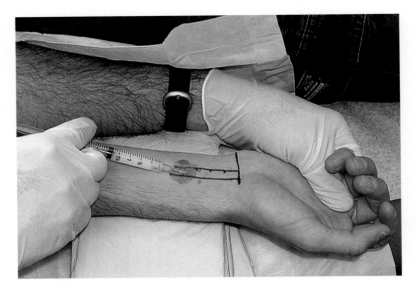

FIGURE 4   ●   Right carpal tunnel injection

4. If any pain, paresthesias, or numbness results, withdraw the needle slightly and redirect the needle tip using a slightly different angle.
5. When the needle has been fully inserted, slowly deposit the steroid solution as a bolus around the median nerve.
6. Inject the steroid solution steadily into this area. If increased resistance is encountered advance or withdraw the needle slightly before attempting further injection.
7. Apply a sterile adhesive bandage.
8. Reexamine the hand after 5 minutes to confirm pain relief or the development of numbness in the distribution of the medial nerve from the local anesthetic.

AFTERCARE

- Have the patient avoid further injury.
- Instruct the patient to use a carpal tunnel wrist brace while sleeping to avoid wrist flexion and extension.
- Use NSAIDs, ice, and/or physical therapy as indicated.
- Consider a follow-up examination in 2 weeks.

CPT code: 20526—Injection of carpal tunnel

PEARLS

- This approach is easy to perform and has few side effects.
- Steroid injections into the carpal tunnel may damage the median nerve.
- Warn the patient that the median nerve may be contacted when using this approach. Ask the patient to report any pain or electrical shock sensation. If this occurs, sim-

ply withdraw the needle a few millimeters before continuing to advance the needle using a slightly different path medially or laterally.

- Because the injection is made just proximal to the carpal tunnel, the overlying flexor retinaculum will not be pierced by the needle.

Wrist Joint

Injection of the wrist joint is a relatively uncommon procedure in primary care. Pain and swelling in the wrist may be the result of trauma, osteoarthritis, an infection, or an inflammatory disorder such as rheumatoid arthritis. Occasionally, there will be a small amount of synovial fluid to remove. If there is no fluid to collect, a small-diameter needle is used for corticosteroid injection.

Indications	ICD-9 Code
Wrist pain	719.43
Wrist sprain	842.00
Wrist arthritis	716.94
Wrist osteoarthrosis	715.94

Relevant Anatomy: (Fig. 1)

PATIENT POSITION

- Supine on the examination table.
- The elbow is slightly flexed with neutral positioning of the wrist in pronation.

LANDMARKS

- Identify the area of maximal tenderness and/or swelling over the dorsal aspect of the wrist joint.
- At that site, press firmly with the retracted tip of a ballpoint pen. This indention represents the entry point for the needle.

ANESTHESIA

- Local anesthesia of the skin with topical vapocoolant spray.

EQUIPMENT

- 3-ml syringe
- 10-ml syringe—for optional aspiration
- 25-gauge, 1-inch needle.

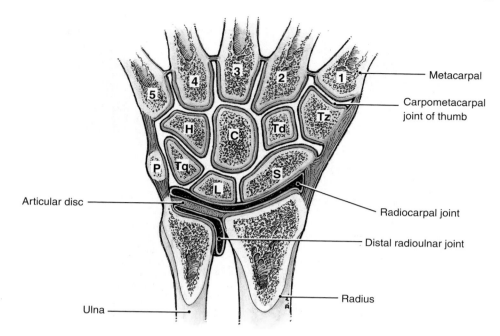

FIGURE 1 ● Right wrist in supination. (Adapted from Agur A, Lee MJ. *Grant's Atlas of Anatomy*, 10th ed. Philadelphia: Lippincott Williams & Wilkins, 1999:510.)

- 20-gauge, 1-inch needle—for optional aspiration
- Hemostat—for optional injection following aspiration
- 0.5 ml of 1% lidocaine without epinephrine
- 0.5 ml of the steroid solution (40 mg of triamcinolone acetonide)
- Alcohol pads
- Betadine pads
- Sterile gauze pads
- Sterile adhesive bandage
- Nonsterile, clean chucks pad

TECHNIQUE

1. Prep the insertion site with alcohol and Betadine.
2. Achieve good topical anesthesia by using vapocoolant spray.
3. Using the no-touch technique, introduce the needle at the insertion site. Advance the needle down into the joint (Fig. 2).
4. If aspirating, withdraw fluid using a 20-gauge, 1-inch needle with a 10-ml syringe, and then inject through the same syringe.
5. If only injecting, use a 25-gauge, 1-inch needle with the 3-ml syringe.
6. If injection following aspiration is elected, grasp the hub of the needle with a hemostat, remove the large syringe from the 20-gauge needle, and then attach the 3-ml syringe filled with the steroid solution.
7. The injected solution should flow smoothly into the space. If increased resistance is encountered, advance or withdraw the needle slightly before attempting further injection.

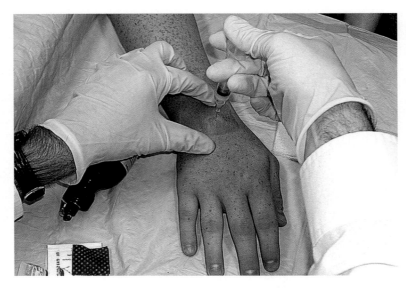

FIGURE 2 ● Right dorsal wrist joint injection

8. Apply a sterile adhesive bandage.
9. Have the patient move the wrist through its full range of motion. This movement distributes the steroid solution throughout the joint.
10. Reexamine the wrist after 5 minutes to confirm pain relief.

AFTERCARE

- Consider use of a wrist brace.
- Have the patient avoid excessive use of the wrist over the next 2 weeks.
- Use NSAIDs, ice, and/or physical therapy as indicated.
- Consider a follow-up examination in 2 weeks.

CPT code: 20605—Arthrocentesis, aspiration, and/or injection of intermediate joint or bursa

PEARLS

- There are many septae that create multiple partitions within the wrist joint complex. Successful administration of corticosteroid involves pinpoint precision and may require multiple injections during the same office visit.
- Work on the dorsal aspect of the wrist. The volar aspect contains the radial artery, median nerve, and ulnar artery. These must all be avoided.
- If multiple injections are performed, do not give more than 1 ml (40 mg of triamcinolone) of the steroid solution to the patient in any single office visit.

de Quervain's Tenosynovitis

Injection of corticosteroids for the treatment of de Quervain's tenosynovitis is a fairly common procedure for primary care physicians. This condition is a stenosing tenosynovitis of the radial aspect of the wrist. The extensor pollicis brevis and abductor pollicis longus tendons run alongside each other and share a common tendon sheath. Overuse movements that require repetitive extension and abduction of the thumb generally cause this condition. However, there may be an underlying inflammatory disorder.

Indications	ICD-9 Code
de Quervain's tenosynovitis	727.04

Relevant Anatomy: (Fig. 1)

PATIENT POSITION

- Supine on the examination table.
- The affected wrist and hand is held in a neutral position. The thumb is directed superiorly midway between between supination and pronation.

LANDMARKS

- Identify tenderness located in the tendon sheath that contains the abductor pollicis longus and the extensor pollicis brevis. The injection point is located directly between these two tendons.
- At that site, press firmly with the retracted tip of a ballpoint pen. This indention represents the entry point for the needle.

ANESTHESIA

- Local anesthesia of the skin with topical vapocoolant spray.

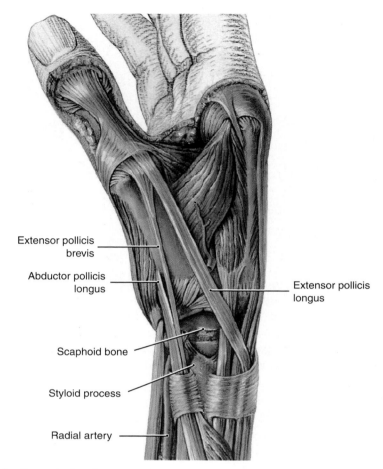

Extensor pollicis
brevis

Abductor pollicis
longus

Extensor pollicis
longus

Scaphoid bone

Styloid process

Radial artery

FIGURE 1 ● Right hand anatomy. (Adapted from Agur A, Lee MJ. *Grant's Atlas of Anatomy*, 10th ed. Philadelphia: Lippincott Williams & Wilkins, 1999:503.)

EQUIPMENT

- 3-ml syringe
- 25-gauge, 1-inch needle
- 0.5 ml of 1% lidocaine without epinephrine
- 0.5 cml of the steroid solution (20 mg of triamcinolone acetonide)
- Alcohol pads
- Betadine pads
- Sterile gauze pads
- Sterile adhesive bandage
- Nonsterile, clean chucks pad

TECHNIQUE

1. Prep the insertion site with alcohol and Betadine.
2. Achieve good topical anesthesia by using vapocoolant spray.

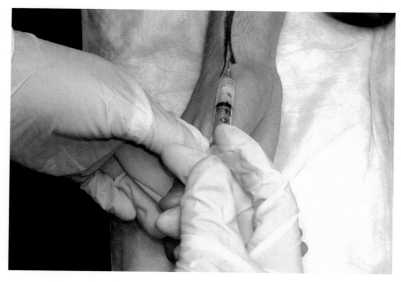

FIGURE 2 ● de Quervain's tenosynovitis injection with landmarks

3. Using the no-touch technique, introduce the needle at the insertion site. Advance the needle slowly and carefully between the two tendons (Fig. 2).
4. Slowly inject the steroid solution steadily into the tendon sheath. A small bulge in the shape of a sausage should develop in the tendon sheath.
5. Apply a sterile adhesive bandage.
6. Reexamine the hand and wrist in 5 minutes to confirm pain relief.

AFTERCARE

- Ensure no excessive wrist flexion or pronation over the next 2 weeks by application of a wrist-thumb spica splint.
- Use NSAIDs, ice, heat, and/or physical therapy as indicated.
- Consider a follow-up examination in 2 weeks.

CPT code: 20550—Injection of single tendon sheath

PEARLS

- The de Quervain's tenosynovitis injection is superficial—especially in thin persons.
- Depositing corticosteroid in the subcutaneous tissues can result in skin atrophy and hypopigmentation. De Quervain's injection is notorious for the development of this complication.
- Avoid the development of a subdermal wheal while performing all injections of corticosteroid solutions.

Ganglion Cyst

Aspiration with a possible corticosteroid injection of wrist ganglion cysts is a common procedure for primary care physicians. Ganglions are thin-walled cysts containing clear, mucinous fluid. They may originate from the wrist joint or tendon sheaths. A common site of occurrence is along the extensor carpi radialis brevis as it passes over the dorsum of the wrist joint. Although most commonly found in the wrist, ganglion cysts may also occur in the foot.

Indications	ICD-9 Code
Ganglion cyst of joint	727.41
Ganglion cyst of tendon sheath	727.42
Ganglion cyst, unspecified	727.43

PATIENT POSITION

- Supine on the examination table.
- If the patient has a ganglion cyst on the dorsal surface of the wrist, the wrist is held in pronation with the wrist in slight flexion. If the ganglion is over the volar aspect, then the wrist is positioned in supination with the wrist in slight extension.

LANDMARKS

- Identify the fluctuant cystic structure over the wrist.
- The injection point is located directly over the cyst.
- At that site, press firmly with the retracted tip of a ballpoint pen. This indention represents the entry point for the needle.

ANESTHESIA

- Local anesthesia of the skin with topical vapocoolant spray.

EQUIPMENT

- 20-ml syringe
- 3-ml syringe—for optional injection

- 18-gauge, 1-inch needle
- Hemostat—for optional injection following aspiration
- 0.25 ml of 1% lidocaine without epinephrine for optional injection
- 0.25 ml of the steroid solution (10 mg of triamcinolone acetonide) for optional injection
- Alcohol pads
- Betadine pads
- Sterile, 2- x 2-inch gauze pads
- Sterile adhesive bandage
- Nonsterile, clean chucks pad

TECHNIQUE

1. Prep the insertion site with alcohol and Betadine.
2. Achieve good topical anesthesia by using vapocoolant spray.
3. Using the no-touch technique, introduce the needle at the insertion site. Advance the needle quickly but carefully into the cyst (Fig. 1).
4. Apply suction with the syringe and withdraw the expected small amount of clear gel (Fig. 2).
5. Withdraw the needle.
6. With gloved fingers, apply firm pressure to the tissues surrounding the punctured cyst. Remove all extruded clear gel with sterile gauze pads (Fig. 3).
7. If injection following aspiration is elected, do not remove the needle. Rather, grasp the hub of the needle with a hemostat, remove the large syringe from the 18-gauge needle, and then attach the 3-ml syringe filled with the steroid solution. In this case, do not attempt to extrude the ganglion fluid after the procedure.
8. If indicated, slowly inject the steroid solution into the ganglion cyst.
9. Apply a sterile adhesive bandage.

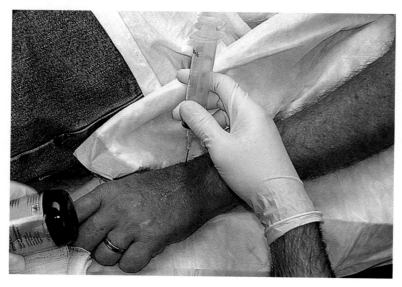

FIGURE 1 ● Left wrist dorsal ganglion cyst aspiration

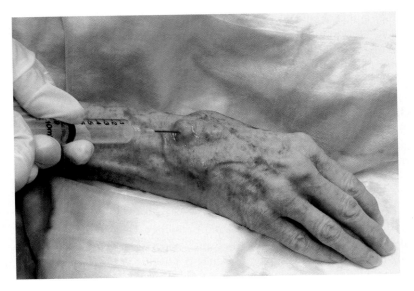

FIGURE 2 ● Multiple ganglion cysts

AFTERCARE

- Consider immobilizing the wrist with a splint for 2 weeks.
- Consider a follow-up examination in 2 weeks.

CPT code: 20550—Injection of ganglion cyst.

  - CPT 2004 gives specific instructions when reporting multiple ganglion cyst aspirations/injections. In this case, the code 20612 is used and the modifier –59 appended.

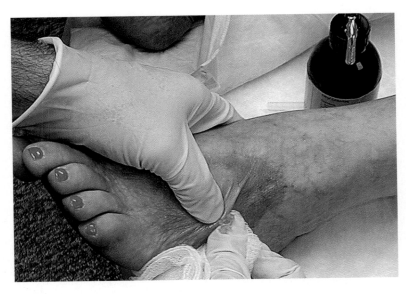

FIGURE 3 ● Expressing contents of foot ganglion cyst

PEARLS

- Use extreme caution when treating ganglion cysts over the volar aspect of the wrist. These commonly involve the area immediately next to the radial nerve. An accidental needlestick of this artery with an 18-gauge needle can have disastrous results.
- Initial treatment of a symptomatic ganglion cyst usually requires only cyst aspiration with manual extrusion of remaining contents.
- Treatment of recurrent cysts may require the injection of a small amount of a corticosteroid.
- Even with proficient technique, ganglion cysts frequently recur and may require surgical referral for definitive management.

First Carpal-metacarpal Joint

The carpal-metacarpal (CMC) joint of the thumb is a relatively common injection site for most primary care physicians. This joint is the most common site of osteoarthritis in the hand. A small-diameter needle is appropriate as this technique is only used to inject steroid solution into the CMC joint. There is no joint effusion to remove.

Indications	ICD-9 Code
Pain of thumb CMC joint	719.44
Arthritis of thumb CMC joint	716.94
Osteoarthrosis of thumb CMC joint	715.94

Relevant Anatomy: (Fig. 1)

PATIENT POSITION

- Lying supine on the examination table.
- The affected wrist and hand is held in a neutral position between supination and pronation.

LANDMARKS

- Locate the CMC joint by palpating the thumb metacarpal bone in a distal to proximal direction. At the proximal aspect of the first metacarpal, there will be tenderness as the examiner's finger passes over, then drops into the CMC joint. This is located between the first metacarpal and the trapezium bone. The patient will report tenderness in this joint.
- The injection point is directly over the CMC joint. At that site, press firmly with the retracted tip of a ballpoint pen. This indention represents the entry point for the needle.

ANESTHESIA

- Local anesthesia of the skin with topical vapocoolant spray.

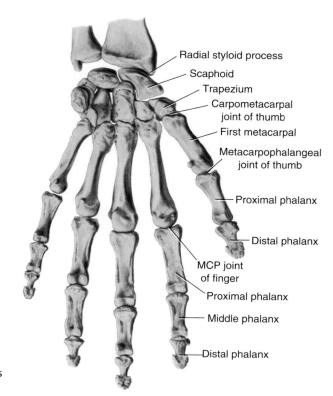

Radial styloid process

Scaphoid

Trapezium

Carpometacarpal
joint of thumb

First metacarpal

Metacarpophalangeal
joint of thumb

Proximal phalanx

Distal phalanx

MCP joint
of finger

Proximal phalanx

Middle phalanx

Distal phalanx

FIGURE 1 ● Right wrist in pronation. (Adapted from Putz R, Pabst R. *Sobotta Atlas of Human Anatomy*, 13th ed. Philadelphia: Lippincott Williams & Wilkins, 2001:180.)

EQUIPMENT

- 3-ml syringe
- 25-gauge, 1-inch needle
- 0.5 ml of 1% lidocaine without epinephrine
- 0.5 ml of the steroid solution (20 mg of triamcinolone acetonide)
- Alcohol pads
- Betadine pads
- Sterile gauze pads
- Sterile adhesive bandage
- Nonsterile, clean chucks pad

TECHNIQUE

1. Prep the insertion site with alcohol and Betadine.
2. Achieve good topical anesthesia by using vapocoolant spray.
3. Using the no-touch technique, introduce the needle at the insertion site. Advance the needle down into the joint (Fig. 2).
4. The injected solution should flow smoothly into the space. If increased resistance is encountered, advance or withdraw the needle slightly before attempting further injection.
5. Apply a sterile adhesive bandage.

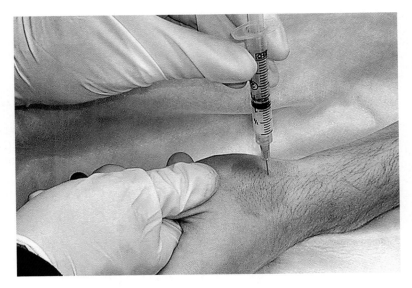

FIGURE 2 ● Left hand, first carpal-metacarpal joint injection

6. Have the patient move the thumb through its full range of motion. This movement distributes the steroid solution throughout the CMC joint.
7. Reexamine the CMC joint after 5 minutes to confirm pain relief.

AFTERCARE

- Have the patient avoid excessive use of the thumb over the next 2 weeks.
- Consider use of a thumb spica splint.
- Use NSAIDs, ice, and/or physical therapy as indicated.
- Consider a follow-up examination in 2 weeks.

CPT code: 20600—Injection of small joint

PEARL

- Applying traction to the thumb in a distal direction as shown in Figure 2 will help open up the joint to accommodate the needle.

Metacarpal-phalangeal Joint

The metacarpal-phalangeal (MCP) joints of the hand are uncommon injection sites for most primary care clinicians. An MCP joint may become inflamed with osteoarthritis, inflammatory, or septic arthritis. A small-diameter needle is appropriate as this technique is only used to inject steroid solution into the MCP joint. There should not be a significant joint effusion to remove in the absence of infection.

Indications	ICD-9 Code
Pain of MCP joint	719.44
Sprain of MCP joint	842.12
Arthritis of MCP joint	716.94
Osteoarthrosis of MCP joint	715.94

PATIENT POSITION

- Lying supine on the examination table.
- The affected wrist and hand is held in a neutral position with the wrist pronated. Ask the patient to make a loose fist.

LANDMARKS

- Locate the affected MCP joint.
- The injection point is directly over the MCP joint.
- The point of entry is located just radial or ulnar to the extensor tendon. At that site, press firmly with the retracted tip of a ballpoint pen. This indention represents the entry point for the needle.

ANESTHESIA

- Local anesthesia of the skin with topical vapocoolant spray.

EQUIPMENT

- 3-ml syringe
- 25-gauge, 1-inch needle
- 0.5 ml of 1% lidocaine without epinephrine

- 0.5 ml of the steroid solution (20 mg of triamcinolone acetonide)
- Alcohol pads
- Betadine pads
- Sterile gauze pads
- Sterile adhesive bandage
- Nonsterile, clean chucks pad

TECHNIQUE

1. Prep the insertion site with alcohol and Betadine.
2. Achieve good topical anesthesia by using vapocoolant spray.
3. Using the no-touch technique, introduce the needle at the insertion site. Advance the needle down into the joint (Fig. 1).
4. The injected solution should flow smoothly into the space. If increased resistance is encountered, advance or withdraw the needle slightly before attempting further injection.
5. Apply a sterile adhesive bandage.
6. Have the patient move the MCP joint through its full range of motion. This movement distributes the steroid solution throughout the joint.
7. Reexamine the MCP joint in 5 minutes to confirm pain relief.

AFTERCARE

- Have the patient avoid excessive use of the affected hand and finger over the next 2 weeks.
- Consider use of a volar wrist splint.
- Use NSAIDs, ice, and/or physical therapy as indicated.
- Consider a follow-up examination in 2 weeks.

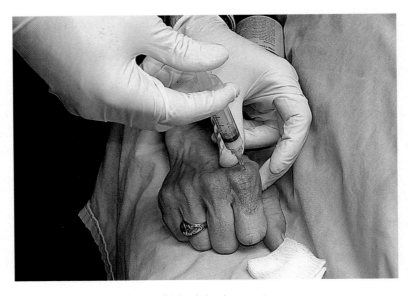

FIGURE 1 ● Metacarpal-phalangeal joint injection

CPT code: 20600—Injection of small joint

PEARLS

- Approach the MCP joint dorsally, but avoid inserting the needle through the extensor tendon.
- Avoid the development of a subdermal wheal during injection. This indicates deposition of steroid solution that may cause localized skin atrophy and hypopigmentation.

Trigger Finger

Trigger finger is the term given for tendinosis of the flexor tendons of the digits. The tendonopathy with nodule formation usually occurs as a result of repetitive compression injury. It is more common in patients with diabetes and rheumatoid arthritis. In this disorder, a nodule forms where the flexor tendon passes over the metacarpal head or, less commonly, the carpal-metacarpal joint of the thumb. With flexion of the digit, the nodule passes over the proximal edge of the A1 pulley of the tendon sheath and becomes entrapped. Although an uncommon procedure for primary care providers, discrete injection of corticosteroids offers an effective, nonsurgical treatment of this condition.

Indications	ICD-9 Code
Trigger finger	727.03

PATIENT POSITION

- Supine on the examination table.
- The affected wrist and hand is held in a neutral position.
- The wrist is fully supinated.

LANDMARKS

- Identify the tender nodule located in the finger flexor tendon and its sheath. This should be at the distal palmar crease.
- The injection point is located just distal to the nodule.
- At that site, press firmly with the retracted tip of a ballpoint pen. This indention represents the entry point for the needle.

ANESTHESIA

- Local anesthesia of the skin with topical vapocoolant spray.

EQUIPMENT

- 3-ml syringe
- 25-gauge, 1-inch needle
- 0.5 ml of 1% lidocaine without epinephrine

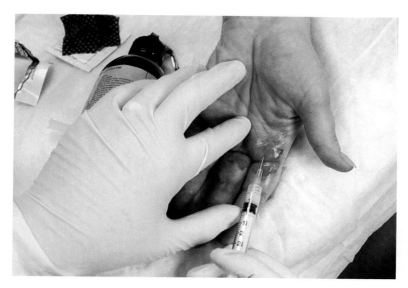

FIGURE 1 ● Trigger finger injection

- 0.5 ml of the steroid solution (20 mg of triamcinolone acetonide)
- Alcohol pads
- Betadine pads
- Sterile gauze pads
- Sterile adhesive bandage
- Nonsterile, clean chucks pad

TECHNIQUE

1. Prep the insertion site with alcohol and Betadine.
2. Achieve good topical anesthesia by using vapocoolant spray.
3. Using the no-touch technique, introduce the needle at the insertion site. Advance the needle at a 45-degree angle. Work slowly and carefully from a distal to proximal direction (Fig. 1).
4. Slowly inject the steroid solution around the nodule into the tendon sheath. A small bulge in the shape of a sausage may develop in the tendon sheath.
5. Apply a sterile adhesive bandage.
6. Reexamine the hand after 5 minutes to confirm pain relief.

AFTERCARE

- Have the patient avoid excessive, repetitive handgrip activities over the next 2 weeks.
- Use NSAIDs, ice, heat, and/or physical therapy as indicated.
- Consider follow-up examination in 2 weeks.

CPT code: 20550—Injection of single tendon sheath

PEARL

- The flexor tendon nodule may be approached from either a distal or proximal direction. It is, however, easier to perform this injection in a distal to proximal direction.

Muscular Trigger Points

Injection of muscular trigger points is a common procedure for primary care physicians. Trigger points are focal areas of muscular ischemia, spasm, and inflammation that can occur anywhere but usually involve the back muscles. They occur most commonly in patients with fibromyalgia/fibromyositis. Although the administration of local cortico-steroid preparation is common, "dry needling" of the lesions may also be effective.

Indications	ICD-9 Code
Tension headache	307.81
Spinal enthesopathy	720.1
Cervicalgia	723.1
Rheumatism unspecified and fibrositis	729.0
Fibromyalgia/fibromyositis and myalgia	729.1
Neuralgia, neuritis, and radiculitis	729.2

PATIENT POSITION

- Lying prone on the examination table.

LANDMARKS

- Identify tender nodules that are usually located in the rhomboid or trapezius muscles.
- The injection point is directly over the nodule(s).
- At these sites, press firmly with the retracted tip of a ballpoint pen. This indention represents the entry point for the needle.

ANESTHESIA

- Usually not necessary, but topical vapocoolant spray may be used.

EQUIPMENT

- 3-ml syringe
- 25-gauge, 1-inch needle
- 1 ml of 1% lidocaine without epinephrine
- 1 ml of the steroid solution (40 mg of triamcinolone acetonide)
- Alcohol pads

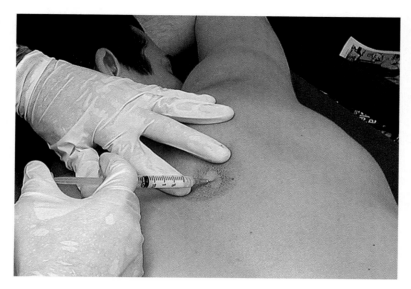

FIGURE 1 ● Trigger point injection

- Betadine pads
- Sterile gauze pads
- Sterile adhesive bandage
- Nonsterile, clean chucks pad

TECHNIQUE

1. Prep the insertion site with alcohol and Betadine.
2. Achieve good topical anesthesia by using vapocoolant spray, if desired.
3. Using the no-touch technique, introduce the needle at the insertion site. Advance the needle slowly and carefully into the nodule (Fig. 1).
4. Slowly inject the steroid solution into the nodule(s). Use a fanning technique to inject the nodule in multiple locations.
5. Apply a sterile adhesive bandage.
6. Reexamine the area of involvement after 5 minutes to confirm pain relief.

AFTERCARE

- Use NSAIDs, ice, heat, and/or physical therapy as indicated.
- Treat the underlying condition.
- Consider a follow-up examination in 2 weeks.

CPT codes

20552—Injection of trigger point(s) in 1–2 muscle groups
20553—Injection of trigger point(s) in 3+ muscle groups

These codes are used only once each session, regardless of the number of injections performed.

PEARL

- Avoid injecting the nodule so deeply as to risk pneumothorax.

Sacroiliac Joint

Inflammation of the sacroiliac (SI) joints is a common condition seen by primary care physicians. Pain of the SI joint may occur after trauma or with inflammatory disorders. The SI joint is a large joint that is easily identified but can be difficult to access.

Indications	ICD-9 Code
SI pain	724.6
SI sprain	846.1
Sacroiliitis	720.2
SI joint arthritis	716.95
SI joint osteoarthrosis	715.95

Relevant Anatomy: (Fig. 1)

PATIENT POSITION

- Lying prone on the examination table.

LANDMARKS

- Identify tenderness over the SI joint.
- The injection point is located directly over the joint(s).
- At this site, press firmly with the retracted tip of a ballpoint pen. This indention represents the entry point for the needle.

ANESTHESIA

- Usually not necessary, but you may use topical vapocoolant spray.

EQUIPMENT

- 3-ml syringe
- 25-gauge, 1-1/2 inch needle

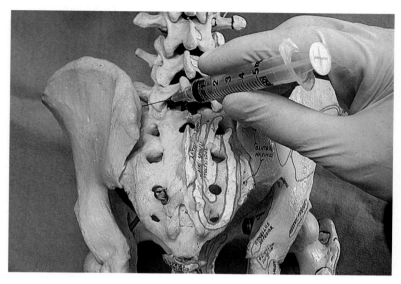

FIGURE 1 ● Sacroiliac anatomy—note the angle of insertion

- 1 ml of 1% lidocaine without epinephrine
- 1 ml of the steroid solution (40 mg of triamcinolone acetonide)
- Alcohol pads
- Betadine pads
- Sterile gauze pads
- Sterile adhesive bandage
- Nonsterile, clean chucks pad

TECHNIQUE

1. Prep the insertion site with alcohol and Betadine.
2. Achieve good topical anesthesia by using vapocoolant spray, if desired.
3. Using the no-touch technique, introduce the needle at the insertion site. Position the needle at a 30-degree angle laterally, relative to the sagital plane, and 15 degrees inferiorly, relative to the transverse plane (Fig. 2).
4. Advance the needle slowly and carefully into the joint.
5. Slowly inject the steroid solution.
6. Reexamine the area of involvement after 5 minutes to confirm pain relief.

AFTERCARE

- Use NSAIDs, ice, and/or physical therapy as indicated.
- Treat the underlying condition.
- Consider a follow-up examination in 2 weeks.

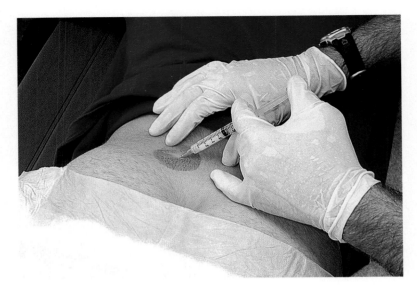

FIGURE 2 ● Sacroiliac joint injection

CPT code: 20610—Arthrocentesis, aspiration, and/or injection of major joint or bursa

PEARL

• Ultrasound guidance may be necessary for correct placement.

Hip

Hip arthritis is a common condition seen in primary care medical practice. Septic arthritis in children is now a rare occurrence since the development of the hemophillus influenza and pneumococcal vaccines. Because of the risk of avascular necrosis of the head of the femur, primary care physicians rarely perform corticosteroid injection of the hip joint.

Indications	ICD-9 Code
Hip pain	719.45
Hip capsulitis	726.5
Hip arthritis	716.95
Hip osteoarthrosis	715.95

Relevant Anatomy: (Fig. 1)

PATIENT POSITION

- Lying on the examination table in the lateral decubitus position on the unaffected hip.

LANDMARKS

- Identify the trochanter of the femur.
- Mark a point 1 cm above the proximal aspect of the femoral trochanter.
- At that site, press firmly with the retracted tip of a ballpoint pen. This indention represents the entry point for the needle.

ANESTHESIA

- Local anesthesia of the skin with topical vapocoolant spray is generally not necessary.

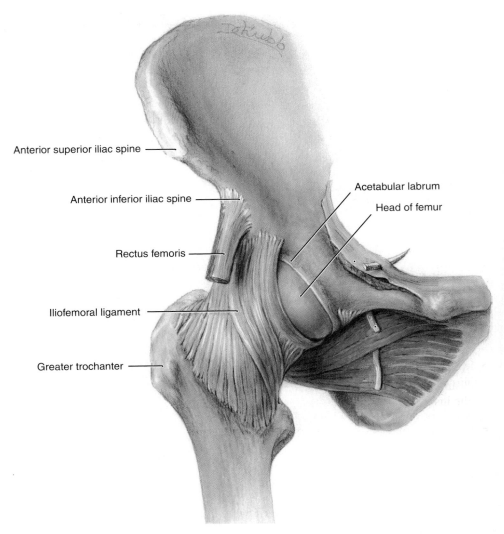

Anterior superior iliac spine

Anterior inferior iliac spine

Rectus femoris

Iliofemoral ligament

Greater trochanter

Acetabular labrum

Head of femur

FIGURE 1 ● Right anterior hip joint. (Adapted from Agur A, Lee MJ. *Grant's Atlas of Anatomy*, 10th ed. Philadelphia: Lippincott Williams & Wilkins, 1999:336.)

EQUIPMENT

- 20-ml syringe—for aspiration
- 3-ml syringe—for injection of corticosteroid/local anesthetic mixture
- 25-gauge, 3-1/2 inch spinal needle—if only injecting
- 20-gauge, 3-1/2 inch spinal needle—for aspiration and injection
- 1 ml of 1% lidocaine without epinephrine
- 1 ml of the steroid solution (40 mg of triamcinolone acetonide)
- Alcohol pads
- Betadine pads
- Sterile gauze pads
- Sterile adhesive bandage
- Nonsterile, clean chucks pad

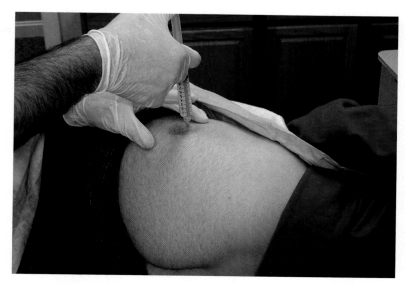

FIGURE 2 ● Hip joint injection—Lateral approach

TECHNIQUE

1. Prep the insertion site with alcohol and Betadine.
2. Achieve good topical anesthesia by using vapocoolant spray.
3. Using the no-touch technique, introduce the 20-gauge spinal needle vertically at the insertion site. Advance the needle touching bone in the hip joint (Fig. 2).
4. Withdraw the needle 1–2 mm.
5. Aspiration should be easily accomplished if an effusion is present.
6. If injection following aspiration is elected, grasp the hub of the needle with a hemostat, remove the large syringe from the 20-gauge spinal needle, and then attach the 10-ml syringe filled with the steroid solution.
7. Inject the volume of the syringe into the hip joint capsule. The injected solution should flow smoothly into the joint space without resistance. If increased resistance is encountered, advance or withdraw the needle slightly before attempting further injection.
8. Apply a sterile adhesive bandage followed by a compressive elastic bandage.
9. Reexamine the area of the hip after 5 minutes to confirm pain relief.

AFTERCARE

- Have the patient avoid excessive weight bearing and hip movement over the next 2 weeks.
- Use NSAIDs and/or physical therapy as indicated.
- Consider a follow-up examination in 2 weeks.

CPT code: 20610—Arthrocentesis, aspiration, and/or injection of major joint or bursa

PEARL

- For large individuals, ultrasound or X-ray fluoroscopic guidance of the spinal needle may be necessary.

Trochanteric Bursitis

Injection of corticosteroids for the treatment of trochanteric bursitis is a common procedure for primary care physicians. This condition is an overuse injury caused by repeated friction of the insertion of the gluteus maximus as it passes over the femoral trochanter. This may occur following repeated stair climbing or walking up an incline. A small-diameter needle is appropriate as there will not be a fluid collection.

Indications	ICD-9 Code
Trochanteric bursitis	726.5

Relevant Anatomy: (Fig. 1)

PATIENT POSITION

- Lying on the examination table in the lateral decubitus position on the unaffected hip.

LANDMARKS

- The point of maximal tenderness over the trochanteric bursa is identified.
- At that site, press firmly with the retracted tip of a ballpoint pen. This indention represents the entry point for the needle.

ANESTHESIA

- Local anesthesia of the skin with topical vapocoolant spray is generally not necessary.

EQUIPMENT

- 3-ml syringe
- 25-gauge, 1-1/2 inch needle
- 1 ml of 1% lidocaine without epinephrine

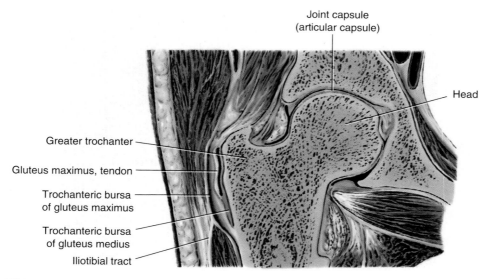

Joint capsule
(articular capsule)

Head

Greater trochanter

Gluteus maximus, tendon

Trochanteric bursa
of gluteus maximus

Trochanteric bursa
of gluteus medius

Iliotibial tract

FIGURE 1 ● Right anterior hip with trochanteric bursa. (Adapted from Putz R, Pabst R. *Sobotta Atlas of Human Anatomy*, 13th ed. Philadelphia: Lippincott Williams & Wilkins, 2001:280.)

- 1 ml of the steroid solution (40 mg of triamcinolone acetonide)
- Alcohol pads
- Betadine pads
- Sterile gauze pads
- Sterile adhesive bandage
- Nonsterile, clean chucks pad

TECHNIQUE

1. Prep the insertion site with alcohol and Betadine.
2. Achieve good topical anesthesia by using vapocoolant spray.
3. Using the no-touch technique, introduce the needle at the insertion site. Advance the needle touching the bone of the femoral trochanter (Fig. 2).
4. Withdraw the needle 1–2 mm.
5. Inject the steroid solution steadily into this area. If increased resistance is encountered advance or withdraw the needle slightly before attempting further injection.
6. Apply a sterile adhesive bandage followed by a compressive elastic bandage.
7. Reexamine the area of the trochanteric bursa after 5 minutes to confirm pain relief.

AFTERCARE

- Have the patient avoid excessive hip movement over the next 2 weeks.
- Use NSAIDs, ice, heat, and/or physical therapy as indicated.
- Consider a follow-up examination in 2 weeks.

CPT code: 20551—Injection of tendon origin or insertion

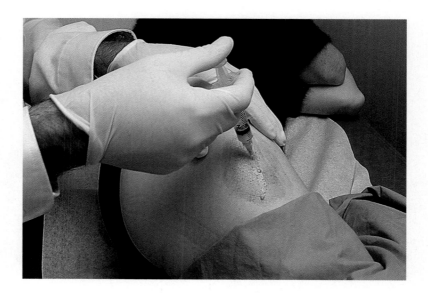

FIGURE 2 ● Trochanteric bursitis injection

PEARL

• Consider fanning this injection to disperse the corticosteroid over a wider area.

Knee—Lateral Suprapatellar Approach

Aspiration and injection of the knee joint is a common procedure for primary care physicians. The suprapatellar approach to the knee joint is the easiest to perform and is well accepted by patients. Because of supine positioning, patients do not see the approaching needle and anxiety is diminished. This approach is considered safe because there are no major arteries or nerves in the immediate path of the needle. Because the injection is done using the suprapatellar approach, it is extraarticular but still within the joint space. As a result, joint fluid can be removed and corticosteroid injected without direct needle injury to the articular cartilage.

Indications	ICD-9 Code
Knee pain	719.46
Knee sprain, unspecified site	844.9
Knee arthritis or arthropathy	716.96
Knee osteoarthrosis, primary	715.16
Knee osteoarthrosis, secondary	715.26

Using local anesthetic, this injection can help the clinician determine the cause of knee pain. After pain has been eliminated as a complicating factor, the knee can be reexamined to assess integrity of the ligaments and menisci.

Relevant Anatomy: (Fig. 1)

PATIENT POSITION

- Lying supine on the examination table with both knees extended.
- The knee may be slightly flexed and supported with folded towels or chucks pads as needed for patient comfort.

LANDMARKS

- Although both the lateral and medial approaches may be used, the preferred approach is from the lateral aspect. This approach affords the operator more room, prevents the patient from inadvertently kicking the clinician with the uninvolved leg, and preserves patient modesty, especially with female patients.

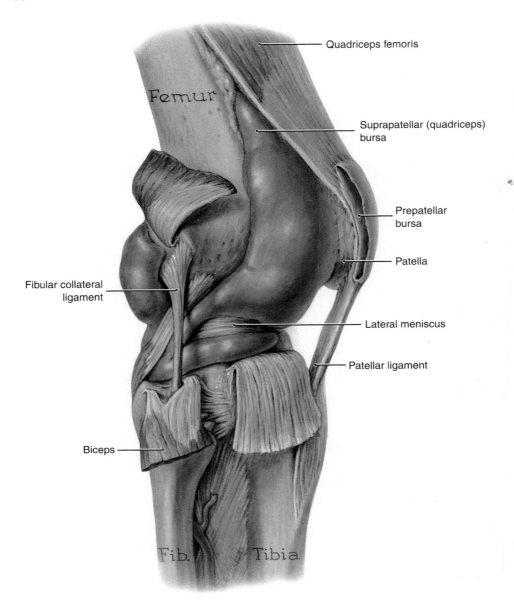

Quadriceps femoris

Femur

Suprapatellar (quadriceps) bursa

Prepatellar bursa

Patella

Fibular collateral ligament

Lateral meniscus

Patellar ligament

Biceps

Fib.   Tibia

FIGURE 1 ● Right lateral knee—distended joint capsule. (Adapted from Agur A, Lee MJ. *Grant's Atlas of Anatomy*, 10th ed. Philadelphia: Lippincott Williams & Wilkins, 1999:358.)

- First, find the superior aspect of the patella.
- Draw a line horizontally one fingerbreadth above the superior margin of the patella (Fig. 2).
- Next, find the posterior edge of the patella and draw a line in a vertical direction.
- Identify the point where these two lines intersect.
- At that site, press firmly with the retracted tip of a ballpoint pen. This indention represents the entry point for the needle.

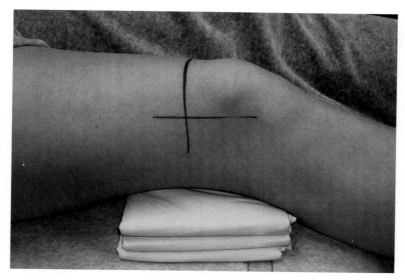

FIGURE 2 ●   Right lateral knee—with lines drawn

ANESTHESIA

- Local anesthesia and vasoconstriction of the skin and soft tissues is obtained using 10 ml of 1% lidocaine with epinephrine.

EQUIPMENT

- 10-ml syringe—for anesthesia
- 20–60-ml syringe—for aspiration
- 10-ml syringe—for injection of the anesthetic-corticosteroid mixture
- 25-gauge, 1-1/2 inch needle—for anesthesia
- 18-gauge, 1-1/2 inch needle—for aspiration
- Hemostat—for optional injection following aspiration
- 10 ml of 1% lidocaine with epinephrine—for local anesthesia
- 8 ml of 1% lidocaine without epinephrine—to dilute the corticosteroid
- 1 ml of the steroid solution (40 mg of triamcinolone acetonide)
- Viscosupplementation agent of choice—if indicated
- Alcohol pads
- Betadine pads
- Sterile gauze pads
- Sterile adhesive bandage
- Nonsterile, clean chucks pad

TECHNIQUE

1. Prep the insertion site with alcohol and Betadine.
2. Using the no-touch technique, introduce the needle for local anesthesia at the insertion site.

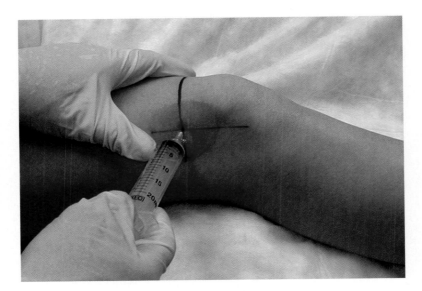

FIGURE 3 ● Right knee injection—lateral suprapatellar approach

3. Next, inject a total of 10 ml of 1% lidocaine with epinephrine to provide adequate local anesthesia. Deposit the anesthetic under the skin, in the soft tissues and over the periostium.
4. When adequate anesthesia is achieved, insert the 18-gauge aspiration needle parallel to the floor and at a right angle to the other two previously drawn skin lines. Advance the needle cautiously while simultaneously applying suction on the syringe (Fig. 3).
5. If the needle touches the anterior aspect of the femur before joint fluid returns in the syringe, then "walk" the needle over the femur until the joint space is entered.

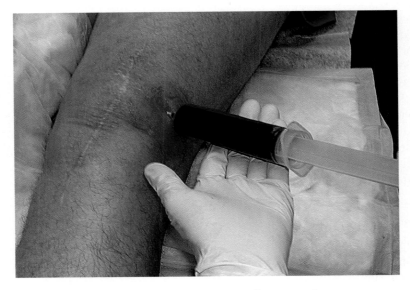

FIGURE 4 ● Right knee aspiration—lateral suprapatellar approach

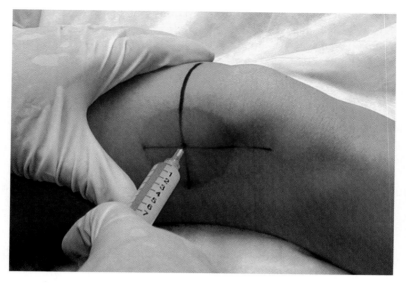

FIGURE 5 ● Bloody aspirate from knee

6. Once the joint space is accessed, fluid will enter the syringe (Fig. 4). Multiple syringes may need to be used to drain all of the synovial fluid.
7. If injection following aspiration is elected, grasp the hub of the needle with a hemostat, remove the large syringe from the 18-gauge needle, and then attach the 10-ml syringe filled with the steroid solution.
8. Inject the volume of the syringe into the knee joint space (Figs. 5 and 6). The injected solution should flow smoothly into the joint space without resistance.
9. Withdraw the needle-syringe combination.
10. Apply a sterile adhesive bandage.

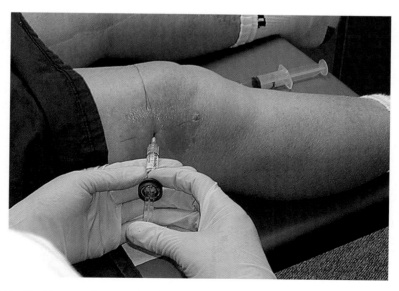

FIGURE 6 ● Viscosupplementation injection

11. Have the patient move the knee through its full range of motion. This movement distributes the steroid solution throughout the knee joint.
12. Reexamine the knee after 5 minutes.

AFTERCARE

- Have the patient avoid excessive use of the affected knee over the next 2 weeks.
- Consider use of a compression knee wrap.
- Use NSAIDs, ice, and/or physical therapy as indicated.
- Consider a follow-up examination in 2 weeks.

CPT code: 20610—Arthrocentesis, aspiration, and/or injection of major joint or bursa

PEARLS

- If the clinician has the unusual situation of experiencing difficulty finding the joint capsule, then either of the following maneuvers can be attempted.
  - Squeeze the interior aspect of the patella and displace it superiorly—thereby shifting joint fluid and filling the superior aspect of the joint space.
  - Redirect the needle in a distal direction to target the undersurface of the patella (Fig. 6). This technique, however, may result in an injury to the patellar cartilage.
- The same approach is used whether the provider is injecting a corticosteroid product or viscosupplementation agent.

Knee—Infrapatellar Approach

Aspiration and injection of the knee joint is a common procedure for primary care physicians. The infrapatellar approach to the knee joint is more difficult to perform than the suprapatellar approach. It is also less well accepted by patients because it may be done with the patient sitting where they can see the approaching needle. There is increased patient anxiety with this procedure, and the patient is at increased risk of injury if he or she develops a vasovagal reaction and falls from the exam table. Because the injection is intraarticular, the knee cartilage over the distal femur can suffer direct damage from the 18-gauge needle.

Indications	ICD-9 Code
Knee pain	719.46
Knee sprain	844.9
Knee arthritis or arthropathy	716.96
Knee osteoarthrosis, primary	715.16
Knee osteoarthrosis, secondary	715.26

Using local anesthetic, this injection can help the clinician determine the cause of knee pain. After pain has been eliminated as a complicating factor, the knee can be re-examined to assess integrity of the ligaments and menisci.

PATIENT POSITION

- Lying supine on the examination table with both knees extended.
- The knee may be slightly flexed and supported with folded towels or chucks pads as needed for patient comfort.
- Alternatively, the patient may be sitting on the examination table or in a wheelchair with both knees flexed at 90 degrees.

LANDMARKS

- Although both the lateral and medial approaches may be used, the preferred approach is from the lateral aspect. This approach prevents the patient inadvertently kicking the clinician with the uninvolved leg and preserves patient modesty, especially with female patients.

- First, locate the patellar tendon.
- Move about 1–2 cm lateral to this tendon. At that point, there normally is a depression.
- Press firmly with the retracted tip of a ballpoint pen. This indention represents the entry point for the needle.

ANESTHESIA

- Local anesthesia and vasoconstriction of the skin and soft tissues is obtained using 2 ml of 1% lidocaine with epinephrine.

EQUIPMENT

- 3-ml syringe—for anesthesia
- 20–60-ml syringe—for aspiration
- 10-ml syringe—for injection of the anesthetic-corticosteroid mixture
- 25-gauge, 1-1/2 inch needle—for anesthesia
- 18-gauge, 1-1/2 inch needle—for aspiration
- Hemostat—for optional injection following aspiration
- 3 ml of 1% lidocaine with epinephrine—for local anesthesia
- 8 ml of 1% lidocaine without epinephrine—to dilute the corticosteroid
- 1 ml of the steroid solution (40 mg of triamcinolone acetonide)
- Viscosupplementation agent of choice—if indicated
- Alcohol pads
- Betadine pads
- Sterile gauze pads
- Sterile adhesive bandage
- Nonsterile, clean chucks pad

TECHNIQUE

1. Prep the insertion site with alcohol and Betadine.
2. Using the no-touch technique, introduce the needle for local anesthesia subcutaneously at the insertion site.
3. Next, inject 3 ml of 1% lidocaine with epinephrine into the skin and subcutaneous tissues to provide adequate local anesthesia and local vasoconstriction.
4. When adequate anesthesia is achieved, insert the 18-gauge aspiration needle into the knee joint angling the needle slightly medially. Advance the needle cautiously while simultaneously applying suction on the syringe.
5. Once the joint space is accessed, fluid will enter the syringe. Multiple syringes may need to be used to drain all of the excess fluid from the joint.
6. If injection following aspiration is elected, grasp the hub of the needle with a hemostat, remove the large syringe from the 18-gauge needle, and then attach the 10-ml syringe filled with the steroid solution.
7. Inject the volume of the syringe into the knee joint space. The injected solution should flow smoothly into the joint space without resistance (Fig. 1).
8. Withdraw the needle-syringe combination.
9. Apply a sterile adhesive bandage.

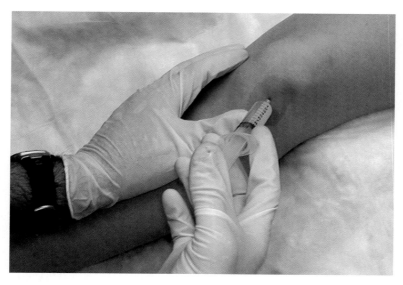

FIGURE 1 ● Left knee injection—lateral infrapatellar approach

10. Have the patient move the knee through its full range of motion. This movement distributes the steroid solution throughout the knee joint.
11. Reexamine the knee after 5 minutes.

AFTERCARE

- Have the patient avoid excessive use of the affected knee over the next 2 weeks.
- Consider use of a compression knee wrap.
- Use NSAIDs, ice, and/or physical therapy as indicated.
- Consider a follow-up examination in 2 weeks.

CPT code: 20610—Arthrocentesis, aspiration, and/or injection of major joint or bursa

PEARLS

- Because of potential direct needle injury to articular cartilage, the infrapatellar approach should only be used in circumstances where the suprapatellar approach cannot be preformed. This may occur in patients with local cellulitis or soft tissue injury or in a patient confined to a wheelchair who cannot be easily moved onto an exam table.
- The same approach is used whether the provider is injecting a corticosteroid product or viscosupplementation agent.

Prepatellar Bursitis

Prepatellar bursitis is a relatively common aspiration and injection site for primary care physicians. Successful aspiration is usually easy because the location of the bursa is readily evident. The subcutaneous prepatellar bursa may become inflamed and accumulate fluid when subjected to repeated excessive pressure or friction. The fluid may consist of blood in acute trauma or thick proteinaceous mucoid fluid after repetitive injury or may be purulent if the bursa is infected. Corticosteroids should never be administered if infectious bursitis is suspected. A large-diameter needle is appropriate as this technique is used to aspirate a large volume of fluid. Occasionally the clinician may elect to inject a steroid solution if the fluid recollects—as long as an infection can be excluded.

Indications	ICD-9 Code
Prepatellar bursitis	726.65

Relevant Anatomy

- See Figure 1 on page 86 (Knee—Lateral Suprapatellar Approach)

PATIENT POSITION

- Lying supine on the examination table with both knees extended.
- The knee may be slightly flexed and supported with folded towels or chucks pads as needed for patient comfort.

LANDMARKS

- The point of maximal fluctuance is identified.
- At that site, press firmly with the retracted tip of a ballpoint pen. This indention represents the entry point for the needle.

ANESTHESIA

- Local anesthesia of the skin is accomplished with topical vapocoolant spray.

EQUIPMENT

- 20-ml syringe
- 3-ml syringe—for optional injection
- 18-gauge, 1-1/2 inch needle
- Hemostat—for optional injection following aspiration
- 1 ml of 1% lidocaine without epinephrine—for optional injection
- 1 ml of the steroid solution (40 mg of triamcinolone acetonide)—for optional injection
- Alcohol pads
- Betadine pads
- Sterile gauze pads
- Sterile adhesive bandage
- Nonsterile, clean chucks pad

TECHNIQUE

1. Prep the insertion site with alcohol and Betadine.
2. Achieve good topical anesthesia by using vapocoolant spray.
3. Using the no-touch technique, introduce the needle at the insertion site. Advance the needle into the center of the bursa.
4. Aspiration should be easily accomplished (Fig. 1). Use multiple syringes if the effusion is large.
5. If injection following aspiration is elected, grasp the hub of the needle with a hemostat, remove the large syringe from the 18-gauge needle, and then attach the 3-ml syringe filled with the steroid solution.
6. Inject the volume of the syringe into the prepatellar bursa space. The injected solution should flow smoothly into the bursa without resistance. If increased resistance is encountered, advance or withdraw the needle slightly before attempting further injection.

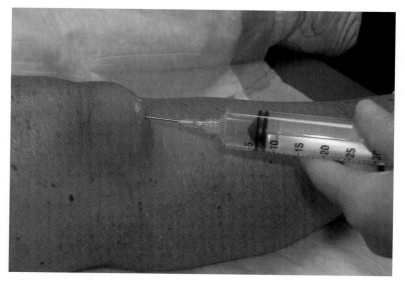

FIGURE 1 ● Prepatellar bursitis aspiration

7. Apply a sterile adhesive bandage followed by a compressive elastic bandage.
8. Reexamine the knee after 5 minutes to confirm symptomatic relief.

AFTERCARE

- Have the patient avoid excessive use of the knee over the next 2 weeks.
- Use NSAIDs, ice, and/or physical therapy as indicated.
- Consider a follow-up examination in 2 weeks.

CPT code: 20605—Aspiration and/or injection of intermediate bursa

PEARLS

- If the prepatellar bursitis is the result of an infection or acute hemorrhagic event, do not follow aspiration with corticosteroid injection.
- Injection of corticosteroid is usually reserved for recurrent bursitis.

Pes Anserine Bursitis

Injection of corticosteroids for the treatment of pes anserine bursitis is a rare procedure for primary care physicians. The pes anserinus is the common insertion for the tendons of the sartorius, gracilis, and semitendinosus muscles. It is located over the medial aspect of the proximal tibia. A small-diameter needle is appropriate as there will not be a fluid collection.

Indications	ICD-9 Code
Pes anserine bursitis	726.61

Relevant Anatomy: (Fig. 1)

PATIENT POSITION

- Lying supine on the examination table with both knees extended.
- The knee may be slightly flexed and supported with folded towels or chucks pads as needed for patient comfort.

LANDMARKS

- The point of maximal tenderness over the proximal medial anterior tibia is identified.
- At that site, press firmly with the retracted tip of a ballpoint pen. This indention represents the entry point for the needle.

ANESTHESIA

Local anesthesia of the skin with topical vapocoolant spray.

EQUIPMENT

- 3-ml syringe
- 25-gauge, 1-inch needle
- 1 ml of 1% lidocaine without epinephrine

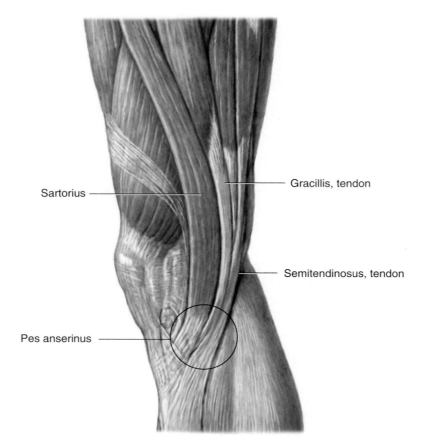

FIGURE 1 ● Right medial knee muscles. (Adapted from Putz R, Pabst R. *Sobotta Atlas of Human Anatomy*, 13th ed. Philadelphia: Lippincott Williams & Wilkins, 2001:328.)

- 1 ml of the steroid solution (40 mg of triamcinolone acetonide)
- Alcohol pads
- Betadine pads
- Sterile gauze pads
- Sterile adhesive bandage
- Nonsterile, clean chucks pad

TECHNIQUE

1. Prep the insertion site with alcohol and Betadine.
2. Achieve good topical anesthesia by using vapocoolant spray.
3. Using the no-touch technique, introduce the needle at the insertion site. Advance the needle to the bone of the proximal medial tibia (Fig. 2).
4. Withdraw the needle 1–2 mm.
5. Inject the steroid solution steadily into this area. If increased resistance is encountered advance or withdraw the needle slightly before attempting further injection.
6. Apply a sterile adhesive bandage followed by a compressive elastic bandage.
7. Reexamine the bursa after 5 minutes to confirm pain relief.

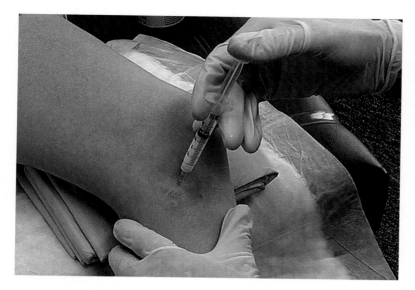

FIGURE 2 ● Left knee pes anserine bursitis injection

AFTERCARE

- Have the patient avoid excessive knee extension and adduction over the next 2 weeks.
- Consider the use of a knee compression wrap.
- Use NSAIDs, ice, heat, and/or physical therapy as indicated.
- Consider a follow-up examination in 2 weeks.

CPT code: 20551—Injection of single tendon origin or insertion

PEARLS

- The pes anserine bursa is superficial; therefore, this injection can be complicated by the development of skin atrophy and hypopigmentation. Avoid the development of a subdermal wheal while injecting the corticosteroid solution.
- Because this is an unusual diagnosis, consider a medial meniscal tear, chondral fracture, or osteonecrosis of the tibia.

Iliotibial Band
Friction Syndrome

Injection of corticosteroids for the treatment of iliotibial band friction syndrome is a fairly common procedure for primary care physicians who care for long-distance runners. This overuse condition occurs as a result of friction of the iliotibial tract as it passes over the lateral femoral condyle. A small-diameter needle is appropriate as there will not be a fluid collection.

Indications	ICD-9 Code
Iliotibial band syndrome	728.89

Relevant Anatomy: (Fig. 1)

PATIENT POSITION

- Lying supine on the examination table with both knees extended.
- The knee may be slightly flexed and supported with folded towels or chucks pads as needed for patient comfort.

LANDMARKS

- The point of maximal tenderness over the lateral femoral condyle is identified.
- At that site, press firmly with the retracted tip of a ballpoint pen. This indention represents the entry point for the needle.

ANESTHESIA

- Local anesthesia of the skin with topical vapocoolant spray.

EQUIPMENT

- 3-ml syringe
- 25-gauge, 1-inch needle
- 1 ml of 1% lidocaine without epinephrine

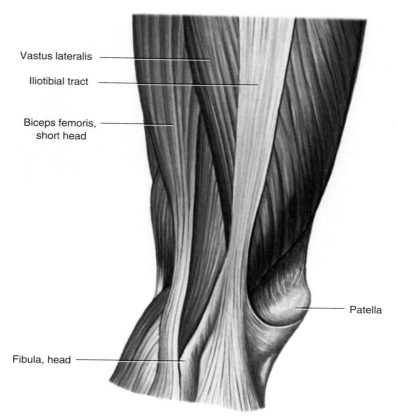

Vastus lateralis

Iliotibial tract

Biceps femoris,
short head

Patella

Fibula, head

FIGURE 1 ● Right lateral knee muscles. (Adapted from Putz R, Pabst R. *Sobotta Atlas of Human Anatomy*, 13th ed. Philadelphia: Lippincott Williams & Wilkins, 2001:316.)

- 1 ml of the steroid solution (40 mg of triamcinolone acetonide)
- Alcohol pads
- Betadine pads
- Sterile gauze pads
- Sterile adhesive bandage
- Nonsterile, clean chucks pad

TECHNIQUE

1. Prep the insertion site with alcohol and Betadine.
2. Achieve good topical anesthesia by using vapocoolant spray.
3. Using the no-touch technique, introduce the needle at the insertion site. Advance the needle through the iliotibial band, and touch the bone of the lateral femoral condyle (Fig. 2).
4. Withdraw the needle 1–2 mm.
5. Inject the steroid solution steadily into this area. If increased resistance is encountered, advance or withdraw the needle slightly before attempting further injection.
6. Apply a sterile adhesive bandage followed by a compressive elastic bandage.
7. Reexamine the lateral aspect of the knee after 5 minutes to confirm pain relief.

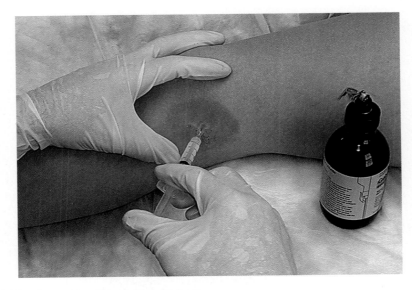

FIGURE 2 ● Left leg iliotibial band injection

AFTERCARE

- Relative rest with avoidance of excessive running for the next 2 weeks.
- Consider the use of a knee compression wrap.
- Have the patient do iliotibial band stretching exercises.
- Use NSAIDs, ice, heat, and/or physical therapy as indicated.
- Consider a follow-up examination in 2 weeks.

CPT code: 20551—Injection of single tendon origin or insertion

PEARLS

- The iliotibial band can be superficial, especially in thin persons. This injection, therefore, can be complicated by the development of skin atrophy and hypopigmentation.
- Avoid the development of a subdermal wheal while injecting the corticosteroid solution.

Ankle Joint

Injection of the ankle joint is fairly uncommon in primary care. Ankle-joint pain may occur following trauma and accompany osteoarthritis, gout, rheumatoid arthritis, or other inflammatory conditions. A small-diameter needle is appropriate as this technique is primarily used to inject steroid solution into the ankle joint. Occasionally, there will be a small amount of joint fluid to be aspirated.

Indications	ICD-9 Code
Ankle pain	719.47
Ankle sprain, unspecified site	845.00
Ankle arthritis	716.97
Ankle osteoarthrosis	715.97

Relevant Anatomy: (Fig. 1)

PATIENT POSITION

- Supine on the examination table.
- The ankle and knee on the affected side are supported by placing rolled towels underneath them.
- The ankle is in a neutral position.

LANDMARKS

- Mark a point just above the talus medial to the tibialis anterior tendon. There is a depression in that area.
- At that site, press firmly with the retracted tip of a ballpoint pen. This indention represents the entry point for the needle.

ANESTHESIA

- Local anesthesia of the skin with topical vapocoolant spray.

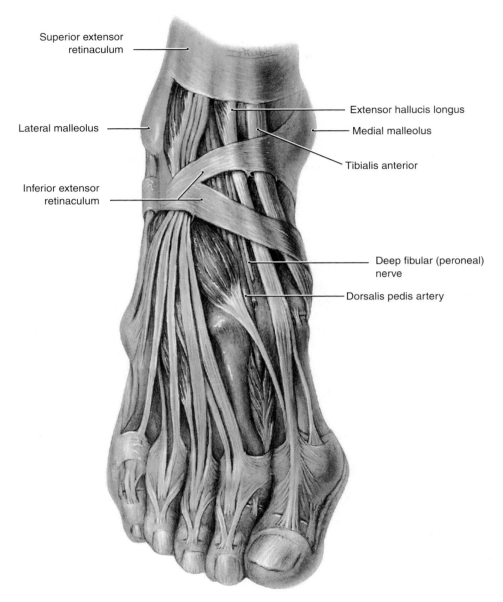

FIGURE 1 ● Right anterior ankle. (Adapted from Agur A, Lee MJ. *Grant's Atlas of Anatomy*, 10th ed. Philadelphia: Lippincott Williams & Wilkins, 1999:368.)

EQUIPMENT

- 20-ml syringe—for optional aspiration
- 3-ml syringe—for optional injection
- 20-gauge, 1-1/2 inch needle—for optional aspiration
- 25-gauge, 1-1/2 inch needle—if not aspirating fluid
- Hemostat—for optional injection following aspiration
- 1 ml of 1% lidocaine without epinephrine
- 1 ml of the steroid solution (40 mg of triamcinolone acetonide)

- Alcohol pads
- Betadine pads
- Sterile gauze pads
- Sterile adhesive bandage
- Nonsterile, clean chucks pad

TECHNIQUE

1. Prep the insertion site with alcohol and Betadine.
2. Achieve good topical anesthesia by using vapocoolant spray.
3. Using the no-touch technique, introduce the needle at the insertion site.
4. Advance the needle into the ankle joint. This places the needle tip between the distal tibia and fibula in the ankle joint (Fig. 2).
5. If aspirating, withdraw fluid using an 18-gauge, 1-1/2 inch needle with the 20-ml syringe.
6. If only injecting corticosteroid solution, use a 25-gauge, 1-1/2 inch needle with the 3-ml syringe.
7. If injection following aspiration is elected, grasp the hub of the needle with a hemostat, remove the large syringe from the 20-gauge needle, and then attach the 3-ml syringe filled with the steroid solution.
8. Inject the volume of the syringe into the ankle joint space. The injected solution should flow smoothly into the joint space without resistance. If increased resistance is encountered, advance or withdraw the needle slightly before attempting further injection.
9. Apply a sterile adhesive bandage.
10. Have the patient move the ankle through its full range of motion. This movement distributes the steroid solution throughout the joint.
11. Reexamine the ankle after 5 minutes to confirm pain relief.

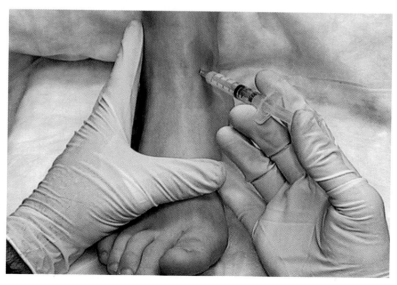

FIGURE 2 ● Right ankle joint injection

AFTERCARE

- Consider use of an ankle brace.
- Have the patient avoid vigorous use of the ankle over the next 2 weeks.
- Use NSAIDs, ice, and/or physical therapy as indicated.
- Consider a follow-up examination in 2 weeks.

CPT code: 20605—Arthrocentesis, aspiration, and/or injection of intermediate joint or bursa

PEARL

- Insert the needle medial to the anterior tibialis tendon to avoid injury to the anterior tibial artery, anterior tibial vein, and peroneal nerve.

Peroneal Tendonitis

Injection of corticosteroids for the treatment of tendonitis of the peroneus brevis tendon is a fairly uncommon procedure for primary care physicians. The peroneus longus and brevis tendons are often injured with inversion ankle sprains. This can cause chronic subluxation of the tendons. Overuse from repeated forceful plantar flexion and resisted foot eversion may also occur.

Indications	ICD-9 Code
Peroneus brevis tendonitis	726.79

Relevant Anatomy: (Fig. 1)

PATIENT POSITION

- Supine on the examination table.
- The ankle and knee on the affected side are supported by placing rolled towels underneath them.
- The ankle is in a neutral position.

LANDMARKS

- With the foot held in a position of active eversion, identify tenderness at and immediately proximal to the head of the fifth metatarsal bone.
- The injection point is located at the insertion of the peroneus brevis tendon on the head of the fifth metatarsal.
- At that location, press firmly with the retracted tip of a ballpoint pen. This indention represents the entry point for the needle.

ANESTHESIA

- Local anesthesia of the skin with topical vapocoolant spray.

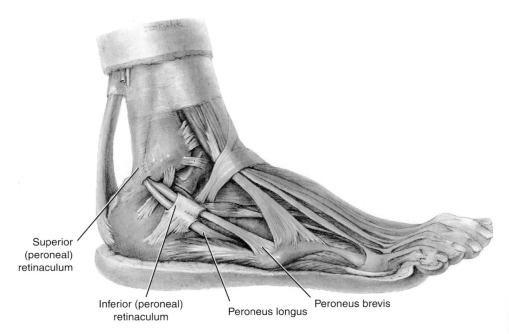

Superior
(peroneal)
retinaculum

Inferior (peroneal)
retinaculum

Peroneus longus

Peroneus brevis

FIGURE 1 ● Right lateral foot. (Adapted from Agur A, Lee MJ. *Grant's Atlas of Anatomy*, 10th ed. Philadelphia: Lippincott Williams & Wilkins, 1999:370.)

EQUIPMENT

- 3-ml syringe
- 25-gauge, 1-inch needle
- 1 ml of 1% lidocaine without epinephrine
- 1 ml of the steroid solution (20 mg of triamcinolone acetonide)
- Alcohol pads
- Betadine pads
- Sterile gauze pads
- Sterile adhesive bandage
- Nonsterile, clean chucks pad

TECHNIQUE

1. Prep the insertion site with alcohol and Betadine.
2. Achieve good topical anesthesia by using vapocoolant spray.
3. Using the no-touch technique, introduce the needle at the insertion site (Fig. 2).
4. Deposit half of the corticosteroid solution at the insertion of the peroneus brevis tendon on the head of the fifth metatarsal.
5. Advance the needle slowly and carefully in a distal direction along the peroneus brevis tendon if treating tendonitis at the insertion of the peroneus brevis on the 5th metacarpal.
6. Advance the needle slowly and carefully in a proximal direction along the peroneus brevis tendon if attempting to access the peroneus brevis and longus tendon sheath. In this case, slowly inject the steroid solution around the tendon. A small bulge in the shape of a sausage may develop in the tendon sheath.

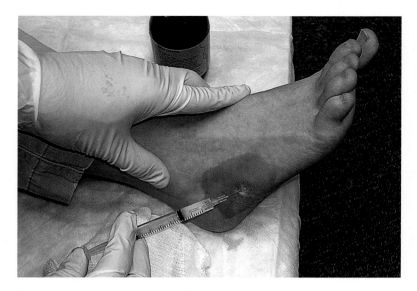

FIGURE 2 ● Injection of right peroneus brevis tendon insertion

7. Apply a sterile adhesive bandage.
8. Reexamine the foot after 5 minutes to confirm pain relief.

AFTERCARE

- Ensure no excessive plantar flexion over the next 2 weeks by use of an ankle-foot orthosis or walking cast.
- Use NSAIDs, ice, heat, and/or physical therapy as indicated.
- Consider a follow-up examination in 2 weeks.

CPT code: 20550—Injection of single tendon sheath

PEARL

- The peroneus brevis tendon is superficial. This injection, therefore, can be complicated by the development of skin atrophy and hypopigmentation. Avoid the development of a subdermal wheal while injecting the corticosteroid solution.

Plantar Fasciitis

Injection of corticosteroids for the treatment of plantar fasciitis is a common procedure for primary care physicians. This condition is a repetitive motion injury to the origin of the plantar aponeurosis at the medial tubercle of the calcaneus. It is usually caused by excessive pronation of the foot, especially in persons with pes planus. The pain associated with this condition is worst when bearing weight after a period of rest.

Indications	ICD-9 Code
Plantar fasciitis	728.71

Relevant Anatomy: (Fig. 1)

PATIENT POSITION

- Supine on the examination table with the hip in full external rotation, knee slightly flexed, and the ankle in a neutral position.
- Alternatively, lying on the examination table on the affected side with the knee slightly flexed and the ankle in a neutral position.

LANDMARKS

- Identify the point of maximum tenderness over the plantar aspect of the foot. This is usually just medial to the midline at the distal edge of the calcaneus.
- Draw a vertical line down the posterior border of the tibia.
- Draw a horizontal line one fingerbreadth above the plantar surface.
- Mark the point at which these two lines intersect over the medial aspect of the foot.
- At that location, press firmly with the retracted tip of a ballpoint pen. This indention represents the entry point for the needle.

ANESTHESIA

- Local anesthesia of the skin with topical vapocoolant spray.

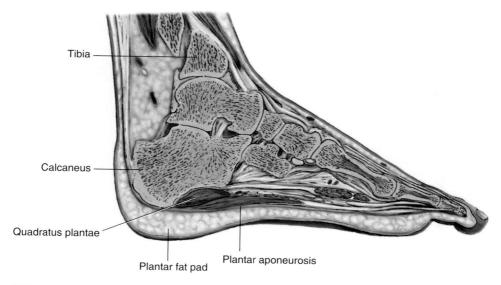

Tibia

Calcaneus

Quadratus plantae

Plantar fat pad

Plantar aponeurosis

FIGURE 1 ● Right foot sagittal section. (Adapted from Putz R, Pabst R. *Sobotta Atlas of Human Anatomy*, 13th ed. Philadelphia: Lippincott Williams & Wilkins, 2001:370.)

EQUIPMENT

- 3-ml syringe
- 25-gauge, 1-1/2 inch needle
- 1 ml of 1% lidocaine without epinephrine
- 1 ml of the steroid solution (20 mg of triamcinolone acetonide)
- Alcohol pads
- Betadine pads
- Sterile gauze pads
- Sterile adhesive bandage
- Nonsterile, clean chucks pad

TECHNIQUE

1. Prep the insertion site with alcohol and Betadine.
2. Achieve good topical anesthesia by using vapocoolant spray.
3. Using the no-touch technique, introduce the needle at the insertion site.
4. Position the needle in a medial-to-lateral direction at a 90-degree angle to the previously drawn lines (Fig. 2).
5. Advance the needle fully, then slowly inject the steroid solution at the origin of the plantar fascia.
6. Apply a sterile adhesive bandage.
7. Encourage the patient to bear weight on the affected foot to distribute the corticosteroid solution.
8. Reexamine the foot after 5 minutes to confirm pain relief.

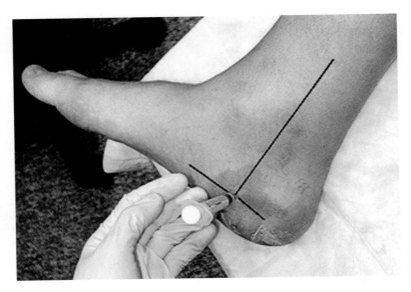

FIGURE 2 ● Right foot plantar fasciitis injection

AFTERCARE

- Use NSAIDs, ice, heat, and/or physical therapy as indicated.
- Instruct the patient to perform heel cord stretching exercises four times a day.
- Have the patient wear proper shoes or orthotics as indicated.
- Consider use of a tension night splint.
- Consider a follow-up examination in 2 weeks.

CPT code: 20550—Injection of aponeurosis

PEARLS

- The plantar fascia injection may be quite painful. This is especially true if the injection is performed through the plantar surface of the foot. The medial approach described above minimizes the pain of this procedure.
- Notice the thickness of the plantar fat pad in the anatomic drawing. The injection should be placed superior to the fat pad to prevent fat atrophy in this critical area.

First Metatarsal Phalangeal Joint

The first metatarsal phalangeal (MTP) joint of the foot is a relatively common aspiration and injection site for primary care physicians. This joint is the one most commonly involved with gout and is frequently affected by osteoarthritis.

Indications	ICD-9 Code
Pain of first MTP joint	719.47
Arthritis of first MTP joint	716.97
Osteoarthrosis of first MTP joint	715.97
Acute gouty arthritis	274.0

Relevant Anatomy: (Fig. 1)

PATIENT POSITION

- Lying supine on the examination table.
- The knee is in full extension.
- The ankle is in a neutral position.

LANDMARKS

- Locate the first MTP joint with simultaneous palpation and flexion/extension of the great toe proximal phalanx. The patient will report tenderness in this joint, and there may be associated erythema and swelling.
- The injection point is directly over the first MTP joint.
- At that site, press firmly with the retracted tip of a ballpoint pen. This indention represents the entry point for the needle.

ANESTHESIA

- Local anesthesia of the skin with topical vapocoolant spray.

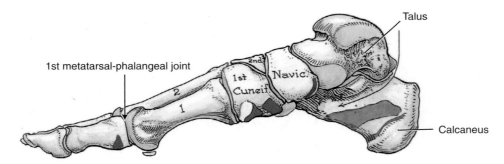

FIGURE 1 ● Right medial foot bony anatomy. (Adapted from Agur A, Lee MJ. *Grant's Atlas of Anatomy*, 10th ed. Philadelphia: Lippincott Williams & Wilkins, 1999:390.)

EQUIPMENT

- 3-ml syringe
- 10-ml syringe—for optional aspiration
- 25-gauge, 1-inch needle
- 20-gauge, 1-inch needle—for optional aspiration
- Hemostat—for optional injection following aspiration
- 0.5 ml of 1% lidocaine without epinephrine
- 0.5 ml of the steroid solution (20 mg of triamcinolone acetonide)
- Alcohol pads
- Betadine pads
- Sterile gauze pads
- Sterile adhesive bandage
- Nonsterile, clean chucks pad

TECHNIQUE

1. Prep the insertion site with alcohol and Betadine.
2. Achieve good topical anesthesia by using vapocoolant spray.
3. Using the no-touch technique, introduce the needle at the insertion site. Advance the needle into the joint space (Fig. 2).
4. If aspirating, withdraw fluid using the 20-gauge, 1-inch needle with a 10-ml syringe.
5. If only injecting corticosteroid solution, use a 25-gauge, 1-inch needle with the 3-ml syringe.
6. If injection following aspiration is elected, grasp the hub of the needle with a hemostat, remove the large syringe from the 20-gauge needle, and then attach the 3-ml syringe filled with the steroid solution.
7. Inject the volume of the syringe into the ankle joint space. The injected solution should flow smoothly into the joint space without resistance. If increased resistance is encountered, advance or withdraw the needle slightly before attempting further injection.
8. Apply a sterile adhesive bandage.
9. Have the patient move the great toe through its full range of motion. This movement distributes the steroid solution throughout the first MTP joint.
10. Reexamine the first MTP joint after 5 minutes to confirm pain relief.

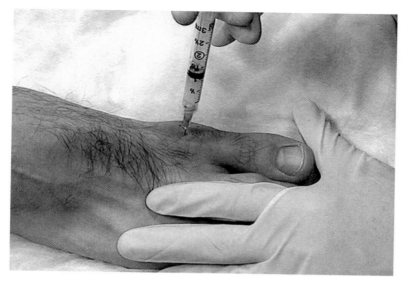

FIGURE 2 ● Right first MTP joint injection

AFTERCARE

- Have the patient avoid excessive movement of the first MTP joint over the next 2 weeks.
- Use NSAIDs, ice, and/or physical therapy as indicated.
- Consider use of an ankle-foot orthosis or wooden-soled shoe.
- Consider a follow-up examination in 2 weeks.

CPT code: 20600—Injection of small joint

PEARLS

- Applying traction to the great toe in a distal direction may help open up the joint to accommodate the needle.

Morton's Interdigital Neuroma

Compression of the interdigital nerves in the foot can result in a painful condition referred to as Morton's neuroma. This is a fairly common condition seen by primary care physicians. The condition is a repetitive compressive injury causing enlargement of the interdigital nerve. Irritation of the neuroma causes symptoms of lancating pain and dysesthesias with weight bearing, especially when wearing shoes with a narrow toe box. Usually the neuroma lies between the third and fourth or the second and third metatarsal heads.

Indications	ICD-9 Code
Morton's neuroma	355.6

Relevant Anatomy: (Fig. 1)

PATIENT POSITION

- Lying supine on the examination table.
- The knee is flexed at 90 degrees.
- The ankle is in a neutral position.

LANDMARKS

- Locate the site of maximum tenderness. This is found between the heads of the metatarsals. The most common site is between the second and third metatarsals.
- The injection point is on the dorsal aspect of the distal foot directly over the area of maximum tenderness. A tender nodule may be identified at this site.
- At that site, press firmly with the retracted tip of a ballpoint pen. This indention represents the entry point for the needle.

ANESTHESIA

- Local anesthesia of the skin with topical vapocoolant spray.

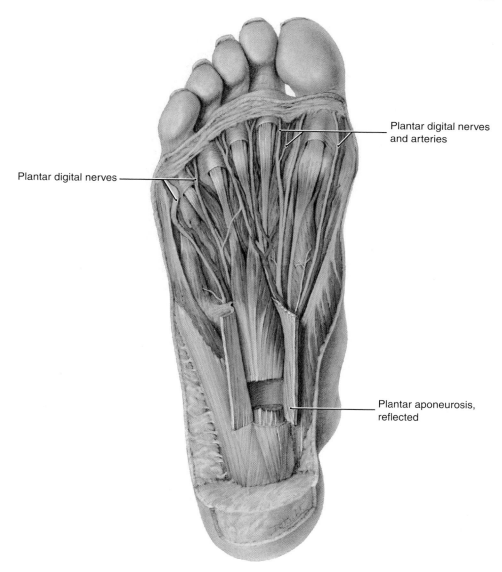

Plantar digital nerves
and arteries

Plantar digital nerves

Plantar aponeurosis,
reflected

FIGURE 1 ● Right foot plantar aspect. (Adapted from Agur A, Lee MJ. *Grant's Atlas of Anatomy*, 10th ed. Philadelphia: Lippincott Williams & Wilkins, 1999:383.)

EQUIPMENT

- 3-ml syringe
- 25-gauge, 1-inch needle
- 0.5 ml of 1% lidocaine without epinephrine
- 0.5 ml of the steroid solution (20 mg of triamcinolone acetonide)
- Alcohol pads
- Betadine pads
- Sterile gauze pads

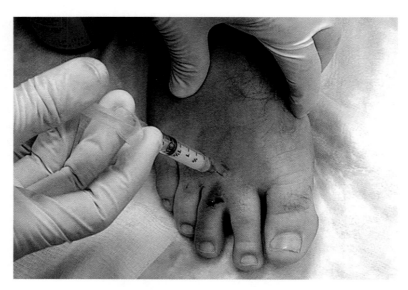

FIGURE 2 ● Morton's neuroma injection

- Sterile adhesive bandage
- Nonsterile, clean chucks pad

TECHNIQUE

1. Prep the insertion site with alcohol and Betadine.
2. Achieve good topical anesthesia by using vapocoolant spray.
3. Using the no-touch technique, introduce the 25-gauge, 1-inch needle at the insertion site.
4. Position the needle at a 90-degree angle to the dorsum of the foot (Fig. 2).
5. Advance the needle between the metatarsal heads.
6. The injected solution should flow smoothly into this area. If increased resistance is encountered, advance or withdraw the needle slightly before attempting further injection.
7. Apply a sterile adhesive bandage.
8. Have the patient apply pressure to the area of injection. This distributes the steroid solution locally.
9. Reexamine the foot after 5 minutes to confirm pain relief.

AFTERCARE

- Have the patient avoid wearing shoes with a narrow toe box.
- Use NSAIDs, ice, and/or physical therapy as indicated.
- Consider metatarsal pads or custom orthotics.
- Consider a follow-up examination in 2 weeks.

CPT code: 64450—Injection, nerve block, therapeutic, other peripheral nerve or branch

Consent for Needle Aspiration and/or Injection

Date: _____

I hereby authorize _____
(Provider's name)

to perform upon _____
(Patient's name)

the following procedure(s): _____

_____

_____

The procedure(s) consists of: _____

_____

_____

_____

_____

(Describe in lay language)

Possible risks associated with the performance of a needle injection/aspiration may include but are not limited to:
Bleeding, Infection, Local pain, Fainting, Allergic reaction, or _____

Possible risks with the use of injected corticosteroids may include but are not limited to:

Feeling flushed	**Flare-up of joint inflammation**
Tendon rupture	**Abnormal thinning of the skin**
Abnormal skin color	**Worsening blood sugars in diabetes**
Impaired immune response	**Disturbance of hormone balance**
Irregular menstrual periods	

The nature of this procedure, methods of diagnosis and/or treatment, and possible alternatives have been explained to me by _____ or his/her associate. I am aware that there are certain risks associated with this procedure and that the practice of medicine and surgery is not an exact science. I acknowledge that no guarantees have been made to me concerning the results of the procedure or it's interpretation.

I certify that I understand the contents of this form.

_____
Signature of patient or authorized representative

_____
Witness

===

IF THE PATIENT IS UNABLE TO CONSENT OR IS A MINOR, COMPLETE THE FOLLOWING:

Patient is a minor, ____ years of age, or is unable to consent because _____
_____ (strike or define).
The undersigned hereby consents to the performance of the above described diagnostic and/or therapeutic procedure on the above patient as well as any tests that are deemed necessary.

                                        _____
                                        Signature of authorized representative

Aspiration and Injection Aftercare Handout

You have just had a procedure performed by: _____

Your diagnosis is: _____

The procedure involved placing a needle into the tissues to:
_____ withdraw fluid from the _____
_____ inject "cortisone" into the _____

Please Follow These Instructions:

Recurring Pain:
Injections are usually done using a local anesthetic such as lidocaine and cortisone. The numbing effect of the lidocaine usually lasts for an hour and then wears off. Improvement in pain from cortisone usually takes 24–48 hours. So, expect the pain to return after an hour and hopefully to go away in 1–2 days.

Rest the Area:
Be careful with the affected area or joint. Usually the injected medicine causes the area to feel numb. Because you may not feel pain, it is very easy to cause further injury to the area. Do not use the area for anything more than mild essential movements for the next 2 weeks.

Watch for Infection:
Although every precaution has been taken to prevent infection, be alert for the following signs: fever above 100 degrees, increased warmth in the area, redness at the injection site, redness moving up the arm or leg, and swelling of the area. If <u>any</u> of these symptoms develop, call this office immediately.

Follow the Directions of Any Checked Boxes:
- ❏ Apply ice to the area every 4 hours for 20 minutes at a time for _____ day(s)
- ❏ Apply a heating pad to the area every 4 hours for 20 minutes at a time for _____ day(s)
- ❏ Apply an elastic compression wrap to the area for _____ day(s)

❑ Perform stretching exercises as instructed
❑ Wear a splint to the area for _____ day(s)
❑ Physical therapy referral
❑ Take the following medicines in addition to your usual medications:

_____

_____

_____

Return to this office in _____ day(s)/week(s) for further evaluation and management of your condition.

References

GENERAL

Baker DG, Schumacher HR Jr. Acute monoarthritis. *N Engl J Med* 1993;329:1013–1020.

Charalambous C, Paschalides C, Sadiq S, et al. Weight bearing following intra-articular steroid injection of the knee: survey of current practice and review of the available evidence. *Rheumatol Int* 2002;22(5):185–187.

Chatham W, Williams G, Moreland L, et al. Intraarticular corticosteroid injections: should we rest the joints? *Arthritis Care Res* 1989 Jun;2(2):70–74.

Cleary AG, Murphy HD, Davidson JE. Intra-articular corticosteroid injections in juvenile idiopathic arthritis. *Arch Dis Child* 2003;88(3):192–196.

Gormley GJ, Corrigan M, Steele WK, et al. Joint and soft tissue injections in the community: questionnaire survey of general practitioners' experiences and attitudes. *Ann Rheum Dis* 2003 Jan;62(1):61–64.

Gormley GJ, Steele WK, Stevenson M, et al. A randomised study of two training programmes for general practitioners in the techniques of shoulder injection. *Ann Rheum Dis* 2003 Oct;62(10):1006–1009.

Green M, Marzo-Ortega H, Wakefield RJ, et al. Predictors of outcome in patients with oligoarthritis: results of a protocol of intraarticular corticosteroids to all clinically active joints. *Arthritis Rheum* 2001;44(5):1177–1183.

Owen DS. Aspiration and injection of joints and soft tissues. In: Ruddy S, Harris ED, Sledge CB, Kelley WN, eds. *Kelley's textbook of rheumatology*, 6th ed. Philadelphia: W.B. Saunders, 2001:583–604.

Paavola M, Kannus P, Jarvinen TA, et al. Treatment of tendon disorders. Is there a role for corticosteroid injection? *Foot Ankle Clin* 2002;7(3):501–513.

Pascual E, Tovar J, Ruiz MT. The ordinary light microscope: an appropriate tool for provisional detection and identification of crystals in synovial fluid. *Ann Rheum Dis* 1989;48:983–985.

Salvarani C, Cantini F, Olivieri I, et al. Corticosteroid injections in polymyalgia rheumatica: a double-blind, prospective, randomized, placebo controlled study. *J Rheumatol* 2000;27(6):1470–1476.

Shmerling RH, Delbanco TL, Tosteson AN, Trentham DE. Synovial fluid tests. What should be ordered? *JAMA* 1990;264:1009–1014.

Simon LS. Therapeutic injection of joints and soft tissues. In: Crofford L, Klippel JH, Stone J, Weyand CM, eds. *Primer on the rheumatic diseases*, 12th ed. Atlanta: Arthritis Foundation, 2001:579–591.

Speed CA. Injection therapies for soft-tissue disorders. *Best Pract Res Clin Rheumatol* 2003;17(1):167–181.

Stratz T, Farber L, Muller W. Local treatment of tendinopathies: a comparison between tropisetron and depot corticosteroids combined with local anesthetics. *Scand J Rheumatol* 2002;31(6):366–370.

Thumboo J, O'Duffy JD. A prospective study of the safety of joint and soft tissue aspiration and injections in patients taking warfarin sodium. *Arth Rheum* 1998(4):736–739.

Vogelgesang SA, Karplus TM, Kreiter CD. An instructional program to facilitate teaching joint/soft-tissue injection and aspiration. *J Gen Intern Med* 2002 Jun;17(6):441–445.

Wang AA, Whitaker E, Hutchinson DT, Coleman DA. Pain levels after injection of corticosteroid to hand and elbow. *Am J Orthop* 2003;32(8):383–385.

Weitoft T, Uddenfeldt P. Importance of synovial fluid aspiration when injecting intra-articular corticosteroids. *Ann Rheum Dis* 2000 Mar;59(3):233–235.

ADVERSE REACTIONS

Acevedo JI, Beskin JL. Complications of plantar fascia rupture associated with corticosteroid injection. *Foot Ankle Int* 1998 Feb;19(2):91–97.

Adleberg JS, Smith GH. Corticosteroid-induced avascular necrosis of the talus. *J Foot Surg* 1991 Jan-Feb;30(1): 66–69.

Basadonna PT, Rucco V, Gasparini D, Onorato A. Plantar fat pad atrophy after corticosteroid injection for an interdigital neuroma: a case report. *Am J Phys Med Rehabil* 1999 May–Jun;78(3):283–285.

Chodoroff G, Honet JC. Cheiralgia paresthetica and linear atrophy as a complication of local steroid injection. *Arch Phys Med Rehabil* 1985 Sep;66(9):637–639.

Comment in: *Am J Sports Med* 1995 Nov–Dec;23(6):778.

Comment in: *Ann Allergy Asthma Immunol* 2003 Oct;91(4):421.

Comment in: *Clin Orthop* 1997 Jan;(334):383–4.

Hofmeister E, Engelhardt S. Necrotizing fasciitis as complication of injection into greater trochanteric bursa. *Am J Orthop* 2001 May;30(5):426–427.

Jansen TL, Van Roon EN. Four cases of a secondary Cushingoid state following local triamcinolone acetonide (Kenacort) injection. *Neth J Med* 2002 Apr;60(3):151–153.

Karsh J, Yang WH. An anaphylactic reaction to intra-articular triamcinolone: a case report and review of the literature. *Ann Allergy Asthma Immunol* 2003 Feb;90(2):254–258.

Leopold SS, Warme WJ, Pettis PD, Shott S. Increased frequency of acute local reaction to intra-articular hylan GF-20 (synvisc) in patients receiving more than one course of treatment. *J Bone Joint Surg Am* 2002 Sep;84-A(9):1619–1623.

Pal B, Morris J. Perceived risks of joint infection following intra-articular corticosteroid injections: a survey of rheumatologists. *Clin Rheumatol* 1999;18(3):264–265.

Reddy PD, Zelicof SB, Ruotolo C, Holder J. Interdigital neuroma. Local cutaneous changes after corticosteroid injection. *Clin Orthop* 1995 Aug;(317):185–187.

Sellman JR. Plantar fascia rupture associated with corticosteroid injection. *Foot Ankle Int* 1994 Jul;15(7):376–381.

Smith AG, Kosygan K, Williams H, Newman RJ. Common extensor tendon rupture following corticosteroid injection for lateral tendinosis of the elbow. *Br J Sports Med* 1999 Dec;33(6):423–424; discussion 424–425.

Stannard JP, Bucknell AL. Rupture of the triceps tendon associated with steroid injections. *Am J Sports Med* 1993 May–Jun;21(3):482–485.

SHOULDER—GENERAL AND SUBACROMIAL SPACE

Arroll B, Goodyear-Smith F. Corticosteroid injections for osteoarthritis of the knee: meta-analysis. *BMJ* 2004; 328:869.

Beals TC, Harryman DT 2nd, Lazarus MD. Useful boundaries of the subacromial bursa. *Arthroscopy* 1998; 14(5):465–470.

Blair B, Rokito AS, Cuomo F, et al. Efficacy of injections of corticosteroids for subacromial impingement syndrome. *J Bone Joint Surg Am* 1996;78(11):1685–1689.

Buchbinder R, Green S, Youd JM. Corticosteroid injections for shoulder pain (Cochrane Review). In: *The Cochrane Library,* Issue 3, 2004. Chichester, UK: John Wiley & Sons, Ltd.

Carette S, Moffet H, Tardif J, et al. Intraarticular corticosteroids, supervised physiotherapy, or a combination of the two in the treatment of adhesive capsulitis of the shoulder: a placebo-controlled trial. *Arthritis Rheum* 2003 Mar;48(3):829–838.

Comment in: *Ann Rheum Dis* 2004 Jan;63(1):111; author reply 111–112.

Comment in: *BMJ* 1998;316(7145):1676–1677, and *BMJ* 1998;316(7145):1676; author reply 1677.

Dacre JE, Beeney N, Scott DL. Injections and physiotherapy for the painful stiff shoulder. *Ann Rheum Dis* 1989;48:322–325.

Green S, Buchbinder R, Glazier R, Forbes A. Interventions for shoulder pain (Cochrane Review). In: *The Cochrane Library*, 2000;(3), Oxford: Update Software.

Green S, Buchbinder R, Glazier R, Forbes A. Systematic review of randomised controlled trials of interventions for painful shoulder: selection criteria, outcome assessment, and efficacy. *BMJ* 1998;316(7128):354–360.

Hay EM, Thomas E, Paterson SM, et al. A pragmatic randomised controlled trial of local corticosteroid injection and physiotherapy for the treatment of new episodes of unilateral shoulder pain in primary care. Ann Rheum Dis. 2003 May;62(5):394–399.

Kosnik J, Shamsa F, Raphael E, et al. Anesthetic methods for reduction of acute shoulder dislocations: a prospective randomized study comparing intraarticular lidocaine with intravenous analgesia and sedation. *Am J Emerg Med* 1999 Oct;17(6):566–570.

Miller SL, Cleeman E, Auerbach J, Flatow EL. Comparison of intra-articular lidocaine and intravenous sedation for reduction of shoulder dislocations: a randomized, prospective study. *J Bone Joint Surg Am* 2002 Dec;84-A(12):2135–2139.

Partington PF, Broome GH. Diagnostic injection around the shoulder: hit and miss? A cadaveric study of injection accuracy. *J Shoulder Elbow Surg* 1998;7(2):147–150.

Plafki C, Steffen R, Willburger RE, Wittenberg RH. Local anaesthetic injection with and without corticosteroids for subacromial impingement syndrome. *Int Orthop* 2000;24(1):40–42.

van der Heijden GJ, van der Windt DA, Kleijnen J, et al. Steroid injections for shoulder disorders: a systematic review of randomized clinical trials. *Br J Gen Pract* 1996;46:309–316.

van der Windt DA; Koes BW; Deville W, et al. Effectiveness of corticosteroid injections vs. physiotherapy for treatment of painful stiff shoulder in primary care: randomized trial. *BMJ* 1998;317(7168):1292–1296.

Winters JC, Jorritsma W, Groenier KH, et al. Treatment of shoulder complaints in general practice: long term results of a randomised, single blind study comparing physiotherapy, manipulation, and corticosteroid injection. *BMJ* 1999;318:1395–1396.

Yamakado K. The targeting accuracy of subacromial injection to the shoulder: an arthrographic evaluation. *Arthroscopy* 2002 Oct;18(8):887-891.

SHOULDER—ADHESIVE CAPSULITIS

Arslan S, Celiker R. Comparison of the efficacy of local corticosteroid injection and physical therapy for the treatment of adhesive capsulitis. *Rheumatol Int* 2001;21:20–23.

Bulgen DY, Binder AI, Hazleman BL, et al. Frozen shoulder: prospective clinical study with an evaluation of three treatment regimens. *Ann Rheum Dis* 1984;43:353–360.

Callinan N, McPherson S, Cleaveland S, et al. Effectiveness of hydroplasty and therapeutic exercise for treatment of frozen shoulder. *J Hand Ther* 2003;16(3):219–224.

Carette S, Moffet H, Tardif J, et al. Intraarticular corticosteroids, supervised physiotherapy, or a combination of the two in the treatment of adhesive capsulitis of the shoulder: a placebo-controlled trial. *Arthritis Rheum* 2003;48(3):829–838.

de Jong BA, Dahmen R, Hogeweg JA, Marti RK. Intra-articular triamcinolone acetonide injection in patients with capsulitis of the shoulder: a comparative study of two dose regimens. *Clin Rehabil* 1998;12:211–2115.

Gam AN, Schydlowsky P, Rossel I, et al. Treatment of "frozen shoulder" with distension and glucorticoid compared with glucorticoid alone. A randomised controlled trial. *Scand J Rheumatol* 1998;27(6):425–430.

Halverson L, Maas R. Shoulder joint capsule distension (hydroplasty): a case series of patients with "frozen shoulders" treated in a primary care office. *J Fam Pract* 2002;51:61–63.

Kivimaki J, Pohjolainen T. Manipulation under anesthesia for frozen shoulder with and without steroid injection. *Arch Phys Med Rehabil* 2001;82(9):1188–1190.

Rovetta G, Monteforte P. Intraarticular injection of sodium hyaluronate plus steroid versus steroid in adhesive capsulitis of the shoulder. *Int J Tissue React* 1998;20(4):125–130.

ACROMIOCLAVICULAR JOINT

Gerber C, Galantay RV, Hersche O. The pattern of pain produced by irritation of the acromioclavicular joint and the subacromial space. *J Shoulder Elbow Surg* 1998;7(4):352–355.

Jacob AK, Sallay PI. Therapeutic efficacy of corticosteroid injections in the acromioclavicular joint. *Biomed Sci Instrum* 1997;34:380–385.

Orchard JW. Benefits and risks of using local anaesthetic for pain relief to allow early return to play in professional football. *Br J Sports Med* 2002;36(3):209–213.

Partington PF, Broome GH. Diagnostic injection around the shoulder: hit and miss? A cadaveric study of injection accuracy. *J Shoulder Elbow Surg* 1998;7(2):147–150.

Shaffer BS. Painful conditions of the acromioclavicular joint. *J Am Acad Orthop Surg* 1999;7(3):176–188.

Strobel K, Pfirrmann CW, Zanetti M, et al. MRI features of the acromioclavicular joint that predict pain relief from intraarticular injection. *AJR Am J Roentgenol* 2003;181(3):755–760.

STERNOCLAVICULAR JOINT

Boehme MW, Scherbaum WA, Pfeiffer EF. Tietze's syndrome—a chameleon under the thoracic abdominal pain syndrome. *Klin Wochenschr* 1988;66(22):1142–1145.

Doube A, Clarke AK. Symptomatic manubriosternal joint involvement in rheumatoid arthritis. *Ann Rheum Dis* 1989;48(6):516–517.

CUBITAL TUNNEL SYNDROME

Hong CZ, Long HA, Kanakamedala RV, et al. Splinting and local steroid injection for the treatment of ulnar neuropathy at the elbow: clinical and electrophysiological evaluation. *Arch Phys Med Rehabil* 1996;77(6):573–577.

ELBOW

Holdsworth BJ, Clement DA, Rothwell PN. Fractures of the radial head—the benefit of aspiration: a prospective controlled trial. *Injury* 1987;18:44–47.

Wang AA, Whitaker E, Hutchinson DT, Coleman DA. Pain levels after injection of corticosteroid to hand and elbow. *Am J Orthop* 2003;32(8):383–385.

OLECRANON BURSITIS

Pien FD, Ching D, Kim E. Septic bursitis: experience in a community practice. *Orthopedics* 1991;14:981–984.

LATERAL EPICONDYLITIS

Assendelft WJ, Hay EM, Adshead R, Bouter LM. Corticosteroid injections for lateral epicondylitis: a systematic overview. *Br J Gen Pract* 1996;46:209–216.

Hart LE. Corticosteroid injections, physiotherapy, or a wait-and-see policy for lateral epicondylitis? *Clin J Sport Med* 2002;12(6):403–404.

Hay EM, Paterson SM, Lewis M, et al. Pragmatic randomized controlled trial of local corticosteroid injection and naproxen for treatment of lateral epicondylitis of elbow in primary care. *BMJ* 1999;319:964–968.

Korthals-de Bos IB, Smidt N, van Tulder MW, et al. Cost effectiveness of interventions for lateral epicondylitis: results from a ramdomised controlled trial in primary care. *Pharmacoeconomics* 2004;22(3):185–195.

Newcomer KL, Laskowski ER, Idank DM, et al. Corticosteroid injection in early treatment of lateral epicondylitis. *Clin J Sport Med* 2001;11(4):214–222.

Smidt N, Assendelft WJ, van der Windt DA, et al. Corticosteroid injections for lateral epicondylitis: a systematic review. *Pain* 2002;96(1–2)23–40.

Smidt N, van der Windt DA, Assendelft WJ, et al. Corticosteroid injections, physiotherapy, or a wait-and-see policy for lateral epicondylitis: a randomised controlled trial. *Lancet* 2002;359(9307):657–662.

MEDIAL EPICONDYLITIS

Stahl S, Kaufman T. The efficacy of an injection of steroids for medial epicondylitis: a prospective study of sixty elbows. *J Bone Joint Surg (Am)* 1997 Nov;79(11):1648–1652.

CARPAL TUNNEL SYNDROME

Celiker R, Arslan S, Inanici F. Corticosteroid injection vs. nonsteroidal antiinflammatory drug and splinting in carpal tunnel syndrome. *Am J Phys Med Rehabil* 2002;81(3):182–186.

Dammers JW, Veering MM, Vermeulen M. Injection with methylprednisolone proximal to the carpal tunnel: randomised double blind trial. *BMJ* 1999; 319:884–886.

D'Arcy CA, McGee S. The rational clinical examination. Does this patient have carpal tunnel syndrome? *JAMA* 2000;283:3110–3117.

Katz JN, Simmons BP. Carpal tunnel syndrome. *N Engl J Med* 2002;346:1807–1812.

Marshall S, Tardif G, Ashworth N. Local corticosteroid injection for carpal tunnel syndrome. (Cochrane Review). In: *The Cochrane Library,* Issue 3, 2004. Chichester, UK: John Wiley & Sons, Ltd.

GANGLION CYSTS

Esteban JM, Oertel YC, Mendoza M, Knoll SM. Fine needle aspiration in the treatment of ganglion cysts. *South Med J* 1986;79:691–693.

Oni. J. A. Treatment of ganglia by aspiration alone. *J Hand Surg (Br)* 1992:17B(6): 660.

Richman JA, Gelberman RH, Engber WD, et al. Ganglions of the wrist and digits: results of treatment by aspiration and cyst wall puncture. *J Hand Surg* 1987;12:1041–1043.

Thornburg LE. Ganglions of the hand and wrist. *J Am Acad Orthop Surg* 1999;7:231–238.

Zubowicz, VN. Management of ganglion cysts of the hand by simple aspiration. *J Hand Surg (Am)* 1987; 12A(4):618.

DE QUERVAIN'S TENOSYNOVITIS

Apimonbutr P, Budhraja N. Suprafibrous injection with corticosteroid in de Quervain's disease. *J Med Assoc Thai* 2003;86(3):232–237.

Richie CA 3rd, Briner WW Jr. Corticosteroid injection for treatment of de Quervain's tenosynovitis: a pooled quantitative literature evaluation. *J Am Board Fam Pract* 2003;16(2):102–106.

Sakai N. Selective corticosteroid injection into the extensor pollicis brevis tenosynovium for de Quervain's disease. *Orthopedics* 2002;25(1):68–70.

TRIGGER FINGER

Lambert MA, Morton RJ, Sloan JP. Controlled study of the use of local steroid injection in the treatment of trigger finger and thumb. *J Hand Surg* 1992;17B:69–70.

Marks MR, Gunther SF. Efficacy of cortisone injection in treatment of trigger fingers and thumbs. *J Hand Surg (Am)*1989;14:722–727.

Murphy D, Failla JM, Koniuch MP. Steroid versus placebo injection for trigger finger. *J Hand Surg* 1995;20A: 628–631.

Patel MR, Bassini L. Trigger fingers and thumb: when to splint, inject, or operate. *J Hand Surg (Am)*1992;17: 110–113.

Saldana MJ. Trigger digits: diagnosis and treatment. *J Am Acad Orthop Surg* 2001;9(4):246–252.

TRIGGER POINTS

Fischer AA. New approaches in treatment of myofascial pain. *Phys Med Rehabil Clin North Am* 1997; 8:153–169.

Hong CZ. Lidocaine injection versus dry needling to myofascial trigger point. The importance of the local twitch response. *Am J Phys Med Rehabil* 1994;73:256–263.

Hong CZ, Hsueh TC. Difference in pain relief after trigger point injections in myofascial pain patients with and without fibromyalgia. *Arch Phys Med Rehabil* 1996;77:1161–1166.

Hopwood MB, Abram SE. Factors associated with failure of trigger point injections. *Clin J Pain* 1994;10: 227–234.

Iwama H, Ohmori S, Kaneko T, Watanabe K. Water-diluted local anesthetic for trigger-point injection in chronic myofascial pain syndrome: evaluation of types of local anesthetic and concentrations in water. *Reg Anesth Pain Med* 2001 Jul-Aug;26(4):333–336.

SACROILIAC JOINT

Ebraheim NA, Xu R, Nadaud M, Huntoon M, et al. Sacroiliac joint injection: a cadaveric study. *Am J Orthop* 1997;26(5):338–341.

Luukkainen R, Nissila M, Asikainen E, et al. Periarticular corticosteroid treatment of the sacroiliac joint in patients with seronegative spondylarthropathy. *Clin Exp Rheumatol* 1999;17(1):88–90.

Luukkainen RK, Wennerstrand PV, Kautiainen HH, et al. Efficacy of periarticular corticosteroid treatment of the sacroiliac joint in non-spondylarthropathic patients with chronic low back pain in the region of the sacroiliac joint. *Clin Exp Rheumatol* 2002;20(1):52–54.

Maugars Y, Mathis C, Berthelot JM, et al. Assessment of the efficacy of sacroiliac corticosteroid injections in spondylarthropathies: a double-blind study. *Br J Rheumatol* 1996;35(8):767–770.

Maugars Y, Mathis C, Vilon P, Prost A. Corticosteroid injection of the sacroiliac joint in patients with seronegative spondylarthropathy. *Arthritis Rheum* 1992;35(5):564–568.

TROCHANTERIC BURSITIS

Shbeeb MI, Matteson EL. Trochanteric bursitis (greater trochanter pain syndrome). *Mayo Clin Proc* 1996;71: 565–569.

Shbeeb MI, O'Duffy JD, Michet CJ Jr, et al. Evaluation of glucocorticosteroid injection for the treatment of trochanteric bursitis. *J Rheumatol* 1996;23(12):2104–2106.

KNEE

Charalambous C, Paschalides C, Sadiq S, et al. Weight bearing following intra-articular steroid injection of the knee: survey of current practice and review of the available evidence. *Rheumatol Int* 2002;22(5): 185–187.

Comment in: *J Bone Joint Surg Am* 2003;85-A(12):2481; author reply, 2481.

Jackson DW, Evans NA, Thomas BM. Accuracy of needle placement into the intra-articular space of the knee. *J Bone Joint Surg Am* 2002;84-A(9):1522–1527.

Leopold SS, Redd BB, Warme WJ, et al. Corticosteroid compared with hyaluronic acid injections for the treatment of osteoarthritis of the knee. A prospective, randomized trial. *J Bone Joint Surg Am* 2003;85-A(7):1197–1203.

Ravaud P, Moulinier L, Giraudeau B, et al. Effects of joint lavage and steroid injection in patients with osteoarthritis of the knee: results of a multicenter, randomized, controlled trial. *Arthritis Rheum* 1999; 42(3):475–482.

Ravelli A, Manzoni SM, Viola S, et al. Factors affecting the efficacy of intraarticular corticosteroid injection of knees in juvenile idiopathic arthritis. *J Rheumatol* 2001;28(9):2100–2102.

Smith MD, Wetherall M, Darby T, et al. A randomized placebo-controlled trial of arthroscopic lavage versus lavage plus intra-articular corticosteroids in the management of symptomatic osteoarthritis of the knee. *Rheumatology (Oxford)* 2003;42(12):1477–1485.

VISCOSUPPLEMENTATION

Adams ME, Atkinson MH, Lussier AJ, et al. The role of viscosupplementation with hylan G-F 20 (Synvisc) in the treatment of osteoarthritis of the knee: a Canadian multicenter trial comparing hylan G-F 20 alone, hylan G-F 20 with non-steroidal anti-inflammatory drugs (NSAIDs) and NSAIDs alone. *Osteoarthritis Cart* 1995;3:213–225.

Adams ME, Lussier AJ, Peyron JG. A risk-benefit assessment of injections of hyaluronan and its derivatives in the treatment of osteoarthritis of the knee. *Drug Saf* 2000;23(2):115–130.

Altman RD. Intra-articular sodium hyaluronate in osteoarthritis of the knee. *Semin Arthritis Rheum* 2000;30(2 Suppl 1):11-18.

Altman RD, Moskowitz R. Intraarticular sodium hyaluronate (Hyalgan) in the treatment of patients with osteoarthritis of the knee: a randomized clinical trial. *J Rheumatol* 1998;25:2203–2212 [published erratum appears in *J Rheumatol* 1999;26:1216].

Dahlberg L, Lohmander LS, Ryd L. Intraarticular injections of hyaluronan in patients with cartilage abnormalities and knee pain. A one-year double-blind, placebo-controlled study. *Arthritis Rheum* 1994;37:521–528.

Disla E, Infante R, Fahmy A, et al. Recurrent acute calcium pyrophosphate dihydrate arthritis following intraarticular hyaluronate injection. *Arthritis Rheum* 1999;42:1302–1303.

Evanich JD, Evanich CJ, Wright MB, Rydlewicz JA. Efficacy of intraarticular hyaluronic acid injections in knee osteoarthritis. *Clin Orthop* 2001;(390):173–181.

Henderson EB, Smith EC, Pegley F, Blake DR. Intra-articular injections of 750 kD hyaluronan in the treatment of osteoarthritis: a randomised single centre double-blind placebo-controlled trial of 91 patients demonstrating lack of efficacy. *Ann Rheum Dis* 1994;53:529–534.

Hochberg MC. Role of intra-articular hyaluronic acid preparations in medical management of osteoarthritis of the knee. *Semin Arthritis Rheum* 2000;30(2 Suppl 1):2–10.

Jubb RW, Piva S, Beinat L, et al. A one-year, randomised, placebo (saline) controlled clinical trial of 500–730 kDa sodium hyaluronate (Hyalgan) on the radiological change in osteoarthritis of the knee. *Int J Clin Pract* 2003;57(6):467–474.

Kolarz G, Kotz R, Hochmayer I. Long-term benefits and repeated treatment cycles of intra-articular sodium hyaluronate (Hyalgan) in patients with osteoarthritis of the knee. *Semin Arthritis Rheum* 2003; 32(5):310–319.

Leopold SS, Redd BB, Warme WJ, et al. Corticosteroid compared with hyaluronic acid injections for the treatment of osteoarthritis of the knee. A prospective, randomized trial. *J Bone Joint Surg Am* 2003;85-A(7):1197–1203.

Lohmander LS, Dalen N, Englund G, et al. Intra-articular hyaluronan injections in the treatment of osteoarthritis of the knee: a randomised, double blind, placebo controlled multicentre trial. Hyaluronan Mulicentre Trial Group. *Ann Rheum Dis* 1996;55:424–431.

Pasquali Ronchetti I, Guerra D, Taparelli F, et al. Morphological analysis of knee synovial membrane biopsies from a randomized controlled clinical study comparing the effects of sodium hyaluronate (Hyalgan) and methylprednisolone acetate (Depomedrol) in osteoarthritis. *Rheumatology (Oxford)* 2001;40(2):158–169.

Pleimann JH, Davis WH, Cohen BE, Anderson RB. Viscosupplementation for the arthritic ankle. *Foot Ankle Clin* 2002;7(3):489–494.

Puhl W, Bernau A, Greiling H, et al. Intraarticular sodium hyaluronate in osteoarthritis of the knee: a multicentre double-blind study. *Osteoarthritis Cart* 1993;1:233–241.

Pullman-Mooar S, Mooar P, Sieck M, et al. Are there distinctive inflammatory flares after hylan g-f 20 intra-articular injections? *J Rheumatol* 2002;29(12):2611–2614.

Tanaka N, Sakahashi H, Sato E, , et al. Intra-articular injection of high molecular weight hyaluronan after arthrocentesis as treatment for rheumatoid knees with joint effusion. *Rheumatol Int.* 2002;22(4):151–154.

Toh EM, Prasad PS, Teanby D. Correlating the efficacy of knee viscosupplementation with osteoarthritic changes on roentgenological examination. *Knee* 2002;9(4):321–330.

Wobig M, Bach G, Beks P, et al. The role of elastoviscosity in the efficacy of viscosupplementation for osteoarthritis of the knee: a comparison of hylan G-F 20 and a lower-molecular-weight hyaluronan. *Clin Ther* 1999;21:1549–1562.

Wobig M, Dickhut A, Maier R, Vetter G. Viscosupplementation with hylan G-F 20: a 26-week controlled trial of efficacy and safety in the osteoarthritic knee. *Clin Ther* 1998;20:410–423.

PES ANSERINE BURSITIS

Kang I, Han SW. Anserine bursitis in patients with osteoarthritis of the knee. *South Med J* 2000; 93:207–209.

ILIOTIBIAL BAND SYNDROME

Barber FA, Sutker AN. Iliotibial band syndrome. *Sports Med* 1992;14:144–148.

Holmes JC, Pruitt AL, Whalen NJ. Iliotibial band syndrome in cyclists. *Am J Sports Med* 1993;21: 419–424.

ANKLE AND FOOT

Khoury NJ, el-Khoury GY, Saltzman CL, Brandser EA. Intraarticular foot and ankle injections to identify source of pain before arthrodesis. *AJR Am J Roentgenol* 1996;167:669–673.

Pleimann JH, Davis WH, Cohen BE, Anderson RB. Viscosupplementation for the arthritic ankle. *Foot Ankle Clin* 2002;7(3):489–494.

PLANTAR FASCIITIS

Comment in: *Ann Rheum Dis* 1998;57(12):749–750, and *Ann Rheum Dis* 2001;60(6):639.

Crawford F, Thomson C. Interventions for treating plantar heel pain (Cochrane Review). In: *The Cochrane Library,* Issue 3, 2004. Chichester, UK: John Wiley & Sons, Ltd.

Dasgupta B, Bowles J. Scintigraphic localisation of steroid injection site in plantar fasciitis. *Lancet* 1995; 346(8987):1400–1401.

Kamel M, Kotob H. High frequency ultrasonographic findings in plantar fasciitis and assessment of local steroid injection. *J Rheumatol* 2000;27(9):2139–2141.

Kane D, Greaney T, Bresnihan B, et al. Ultrasound guided injection of recalcitrant plantar fasciitis. *Ann Rheum Dis* 1998;57(6):383–384.

Lemont H, Ammirati KM, Usen N. Plantar fasciitis: a degenerative process (fasciosis) without inflammation. *J Am Podiatr Med Assoc* 2003;93(3):234–237.

Tsai WC, Wang CL, Tang FT, et al. Treatment of proximal plantar fasciitis with ultrasound-guided steroid injection. *Arch Phys Med Rehabil.* 2000;81(10):1416–1421.

METATARSAL PHALANGEAL JOINT

Boxer MC. Osteoarthritis involving the metatarsophalangeal joints and management of metatarsophalangeal joint pain via injection therapy. *Clin Podiatr Med Surg* 1994;11:125–132.

Mizel MS, Michelson JD. Nonsurgical treatment of monarticular nontraumatic synovitis of the second metatarsophalangeal joint. *Foot Ankle Int* 1997;18:424–426.

Scott PM. Arthrocentesis to diagnose and treat acute gouty arthritis in the great toe. *JAAPA* 2000;13(10):93–96.

Solan MC, Calder JD, Bendall SP. Manipulation and injection for hallux rigidus. Is it worthwhile? *J Bone Joint Surg (Br)* 2001;83:706–708.

MORTON'S INTERDIGITAL NEUROMA

Bennett GL, Graham CE, Mauldin DM. Morton's interdigital neuroma: a comprehensive treatment protocol. *Foot Ankle Int* 1995;16(12):760–763.

Rasmussen MR, Kitaoka HB, Patzer GL. Nonoperative treatment of plantar interdigital neuroma with a single corticosteroid injection. *Clin Orthop* 1996;(326):188–193.

Wu KK. Morton's interdigital neuroma: a clinical review of its etiology, treatment, and results. *J Foot Ankle Surg* 1996;35:112–119.

Index